Praise for *The*

John Daugherty shines light on how symptoms are better seen as information or gateways into their emotional—and often traumatic—causes. His book includes background to the bodymind tradition and describes in friendly and accessible ways a number of self-help strategies that any of us can learn and practice, both to heal and to maintain health. I highly recommend Dr. Daugherty's work and await his future publications.

—**John Hartung**
Principal, Colorado Center for Alternative Psychology

The Health Code is the perfect blend of emotional, mental, and energetic healing. Dr. Daugherty's intimate insight into the principles and tools he used to beat cancer are inspiring and educational.

—**Jeremy W. Greenfield**
Chief Brand Officer @ Popl

John is a special type of health care practitioner— a true healer. He is someone interested in the complexity of your wellbeing and how your emotions are related to dysfunctional manifestations in your body. I urge you to take time to slowly read and digest this book as a starting point for optimizing your heath and the health of those who may be under your care.

—**Laurence Berarducci MD FACC**
Director of Outpatient Heart Failure Clinic, Pueblo, CO

Written from a place of deep authentic experience as a seasoned professional, this book is a comprehensive resource for practitioners and those on their individual journey of self-care. The Health Code weaves together ancient philosophy with cutting edge research, case studies and theoretical frameworks providing an invaluable resource we look forward to highly recommending in our private practices.

—**John & Lisa Matthews**
Directors of IllumineNation
Coaching Mentoring Leadership Yoga, Melbourne, Australia

Dr. Daugherty, backed by decades of hands-on experience and keen insight into his clients' physical complaints and their underlying causes, has presented to practitioners a thorough process of assessing and treating these conditions. The book is a guide that belongs in the armamentarium of every practitioner of the healing arts.

—**Dr. Michael Brown, MD, Neurosurgeon**

Dr. John Daugherty is a master at teaching how to listen to the "unspoken voice in the body" that whispers to us the stories of our past that manifest as illness and injury. With Dr. Daugherty as our guide, the Healing Code is a tool for deep listening to these disempowering stories held in our inner terrain so that we may heal and transform.

—Alexandra DelGaudio
Re-memberment Guide for Stones Stars and Story

THE HEALTH
CODE

ALIGNING THE MIND AND BODY
FOR OPTIMAL WELLNESS

Dr. Shank

This a gift we don't know each other but I'm aware of your great reputation, Enjoy the book!

John Daugherty

THE HEALTH CODE
Aligning the Mind and Body for Optimal Wellness

Edited by Heather M. Hilliard and Shauna Hardy
Cover design by Melissa Williams Design
Interior formatting by Melissa Williams Design and A.J. Reid Creative

For permissions contact:

Quantum Living Press
An imprint of GracePoint Publishing

GracePoint Matrix, LLC
322 N Tejon St. #207
Colorado Springs CO 80903
www.GracePointMatrix.com
Email: Admin@GracePointMatrix.com
SAN # 991-6032

Library of Congress Number: 2020944467

ISBN-13: (Paperback): 978-1-951694-09-8

Ebook: 978-1-951694-30-2

Books may be purchased for educational, business, or sales promotional use.

For bulk order requests and price schedule contact:
Orders@GracePointPublishing.com

Printed in the United States of America

Download your book resources here: TheHealthcodebook.com

Disclaimer

This book's intended purpose is not to substitute the medical advice of a physician or qualified therapist. The reader should regularly consult a physician in matters relating to his/her health and particularly with respect to any symptoms that may require diagnosis or medical attention.

Essential oil warning:

Using undiluted essential oils directly on the skin or in nasal passages may burn or irritate sensitive skin. Some people may develop skin rashes or discover allergic reactions. Administering essential oils improperly may cause adverse effects and some essential oils are poisonous when absorbed through skin exposure.

Certain essential oils in the citrus family (to include bergamot) may cause phototoxicity if used before sun exposure. Always take care to limit sun exposure when using oils in this family.

THE HEALTH
CODE

ALIGNING THE MIND AND BODY
FOR OPTIMAL WELLNESS

DR. JOHN DAUGHERTY

Table of Contents

Foreword

Whether you are a practitioner in the healing arts or a seeker along the path of your own individual exploration and transformation, you will now be introduced to some healing codes that will align your mind-body and help you achieve optimal wellness. This book will help you as a practitioner to expand your own awareness of the magnificent healing potential of the physical life that you have, literally, at your fingertips. It is through these pages that you will now be given a new way to hear the underlying factors and causes of your, or your client's pain or suffering. You will learn to become a more empathic listener when face-to-face with the individual souls sitting in front of you during your healing work.

As a seeker or healer or both, you will learn more about yourself and the power you have to transcend whatever illness or challenge you or your clients may be facing now or in the future. Your body is a barometer of the quality of your life's alignment (or misalignment) with your inspired mission or soul's purpose. Knowing how to decipher the codes your body is giving you when it experiences pain or other symptoms not only facilitates physical alignment but catalyzes the possibility that healing your pain sets the stage for the expansion of our soul's journey.

Symptoms arise in your body as a way for you to evolve along your journey in life. You can use your physical symptoms and pain as codes to unlock the door to your individual growth that benefits your mental, emotional, and physical well-being. These symptoms and their codes can come in a sequence and help you understand your subconscious story lines, the story lines that often keep you stuck in patterns that 'fail' to illuminate your true potential for your greatness.

You are possibly living out stories that you didn't even consciously choose. You may have adopted different parts of your stories from your family dynamics, your traumas, your beliefs, and your perceptions and even injected some from those you have subordinated to. You probably began crafting your individual narratives at a tender age, without even being aware of it. Your imprinting and conditioning from your families of origin, from your own individual experiences—even from your ancestral lineage—have probably been running your life for many years.

This book gives you the healing codes to understand how to transcend such story based illnesses and awaken wellness through reflection and meaning, through rewriting your individual narratives that have caused you to make choices that reflect less than who you truly are—and less than what you are worthy of.

The gift these codes will bring to your clients will be breaking them free from old limiting patterns and giving them a new narrative that impacts every facet of their lives. It's beautifully surprising when the work you do as a practitioner not only heals physical pain, but helps your clients align with healthier relationships, a deeper spiritual connection, greater capacities for abundance, and a deeper awareness of their authentic selves.

The information within this book is an elegant blend of the eastern and western, ancient and modern, physical and subtle, essential wisdom of mind and body for guided healing. Like a pass code that opens a secure doorway, you can utilize the codes to unlock your ability to heal your or your client's old trauma and for you and they to become aware of the feelings or emotions that stimulate illness based thoughts within your and their minds.

Without a more reflective awareness, your thoughts can generate more of the same feelings keeping you trapped in a cycle of repetitive thoughts and emotions that keep you in your habitual behaviors. Because your mind, an artifact of your neurobiology, does such a remarkable job of making our thoughts automatic, often you have no choice but to experience a crisis in your body to bring to your awareness the patterns that make your life so difficult.

This book explores how your feelings and emotions are part of your healing cycle, helping you to release your stored misperceptions or narratives. This is a part of healing many practitioners resist since they are often trained to look at the body as a separate thing from the emotions and the mentally inspiring soul.

Since your emotions are often held in the tissues of your body, they generate the chemistry of the pain and inflammation that creates your physical body's symptoms. As you release or transcend the emotions, you learn to break through the cycle of these habitual behaviors. This affords you an opportunity to change the way you think and change the meanings you hold about core experiences, stories, and beliefs you've been holding in the body for often a lifetime.

If you change the way you think, you unleash the potential to heal and to change your behavior. Disrupting your old patterns, rewriting your old limiting narratives, and understanding the relationship between these thought forms and your emotions and body, give you access to the combination that can break the lock on the door of your limited beliefs, attitude, perceptions and behaviors. As you read this book you will all be inspired by John's touching stories of what appear to be "miraculous" healings. What John will show you in this book is that tapping into the power of the miraculous healing isn't really so "miraculous". Healing at the depth that John teaches in this book facilitates clearing and aligning on a deep level, helping you or your client break free from the patterns of the past and deepening your and their resiliency and ability to continue to access high levels of well-being, inner fulfillment, and health.

In this book you will learn a systematic approach to consistently producing seemingly miraculous outcomes for your clients. You will understand that you are capable of experiencing such healing miracles in a predictable and consistent way.

Renewal is built into the very fabric of your body. In truth, degeneration and disease are the exception, not the norm. Even though most individuals accept aging, degeneration, and disease as a "part of life", once you understand how your body renews itself through wisely listening to your symptoms and opening to the many ways you can heal, you can start to harness the emotional and physiological processes intentionally, which creates the space in your life to reflect, redirect, and move your energy into thriving rather than surviving.

Read these pages and you will expand your awareness, intuition, and your capacity to help your clients facilitate their own spontaneous healings. Through these pages you will learn that you have access to a deeper degree of insight and wisdom for your clients that can help you more effectively and efficiently ease their pain and suffering.

It is my hope that in reading this book you will remember the whispering of your inner knowing of your own body and help your clients do the same, that you will deepen your skillset as a healer and that miracles will become a daily part of your now inspired practice.

Dr. John Demartini
International best-selling author of *The Values Factor*
drdemartini.com

A Note from the Author

My life experience has been a constant and continuous quest for growth and understanding of the universal laws and principles and how they interact with human values, behaviors, health and wellness. I have studied health, healing and human behavior from a bio-energetic wellness perspective creating a confluence of physical, mental, emotional and spiritual energies and how they influence the quality of our life experience. My love is learning, teaching, speaking and sharing strategies for experiencing your truly authentic self, the inspired self. This experience allows you to open to your greatest potential with the possibilities that are available to you right now. I have 40 years' experience in healing, workshops, coaching and sharing.

Now the practical and somewhat boring information about who I am. I have been practicing Chiropractic for 35+ years, and in that time, I have studied and explored multiple methods and processes of healing. I trained and practice as a Chiropractic Physician, although most of my clients and patients just call me a healer. I am grateful for that designation, because healing entails many different aspects of who I hope to be in the world. I have advanced studies in Bio-Energy medicine, Functional and Integrative medicine, as well as being a Board-Certified Chiropractic Sports Physician. I have studied various personal Coaching methods and have trained in many human behavior trainings, such as the Hendricks Institute, Psych K, Neuro-Emotional and Somato-Emotional Therapies.

All of this said, through years of study and practice, I have developed many of my own approaches to health and healing. These methods encompass the ability to create change in physical, mental, emotional and behavioral aspects of each and every patient. These methods have been brought out in this book, and my hope is that you as a reader will benefit from what you learn here. If you are a health practitioner, my hope is that you will find a way to utilize the information in this book to help clients and patients in your own practices. That would be the ultimate honor to have shared something that would help someone, somewhere that I have never even met in my life, but was able to share the energy of healing through another practitioner.

I would like to direct you to more information about me on my website drjohndaugherty.com which gives you my intentions and my commitment to serving my community. Please take some time to browse around.

My hope for you is that you find healing, transformation, and the best version of yourself expressed in the world.

Dr. John Daugherty

Preface

Thirty-five years ago, I was a young doctor and was not aware of the earlier works of great scientist-healers like Dr. Wilhelm Reich, MD, Dr. Ida Rolf, MD, Dr. Peter Levine, PhD, and others whom I have come to know and study. I came up in the profession with the great minds of Dr. George Goodheart, DC, Dr. Alan G. Beardall, and figured my way through practice and patient care alongside Dr. Scott Walker, DC, Dr. John Brimhall, DC and Dr. Ted Morter, DC; all incredibly dedicated doctors and innovators. Their scientific research and clinical experience has helped me for nearly three decades to open my mind as a healer and practitioner. I originally began writing this book twenty years ago, as we were all developing our healing approaches on a daily basis with our patients. Even while all of these individuals were applying the scientific works of our time and putting our focus on healing varying aspects of the human condition, it was almost all theory then. Though these works clinically created great outcomes, it took testing and time to bring this book together in a sensible way using constantly evolving science and clinical methods. The thought-leaders in the early 1980's were just beginning to speak to each other about their discoveries, which made it difficult to develop a healing protocol that would be applied in practice as well as in life.

In meeting my own need for learning, I was able to bring others' studies and my own clinical experience into a collaboration of material for my own personal benefit as well as to the benefit of others. Three decades later, there is greater cooperation between practitioners as well as within fields to bring together the work of many who have made huge contributions to the understanding of how the mind, body, and emotions interact. There is greater focus on what is useful at helping heal the traumas that challenge us in our lives.

We now have the ability to utilize the power of our minds, emotions, and bodies in ways we know intuitively and scientifically work to improve our lives. Evolution of techniques and combined therapies as practitioners and being able to help patients apply exercises and focused skills around self-care and self-healing methods have improved our ability to address the trauma within ourselves. We can use these methods to enhance our lives, our performance, and our health.

The most important thing about your journey using the information in this book is not just the success of healing an issue, pain or symptom. What is most important is crafting your personal approach with an open-minded perspective. These concepts and ways of thinking lead to your own process of self-inquiry and healing as a journey of discovery. The principles and tools in this book are a helpful engagement of self-care practice and self-healing. It can help you with challenges and other struggles you are having in your own life, whether you are dealing with cancer, other diseases, or unresolved trauma. As healers and practitioners, you can easily apply these methods and approaches to your own patients and integrate a broader skill set to your professional development.

As these concepts and principles worked for me, I believe that others could benefit from them as well. I feel that energy integration is a missing part of most medical intervention. The new science on how the body is energetically organized, and how we as healers can influence these subtle energies, is a powerful tool available for those who want to radically change the lives of others as well as their own. We have the influence from our colleagues and teachers: Dr. Carol McMakin, DC, Dr. John F. Demartini, Dr. Louisa Williams, DC, ND, Dr. George Gonzalez, DC, Dr. Richard Gerber, MD and many more who are changing the way we approach healing. They are developing and utilizing many different approaches of energy medicine to improve the lives of doctors and patients. Through their generosity of sharing what they have learned, they are educating a tribe of doctors that are benefiting and changing the lives of millions around the globe. I hope my small contribution through this book will bring more awareness to healers about the work of others and add to the advancement of their skills. My desire is that this book will create a tribe of people who are in the mainstream and complementary healing arts to be more open-minded to the new science of emotional, mental, and energetic healing that is now available. My hope is also that the collaboration of your tribe of healers, both medical and complementary practitioners, help you take the responsibility to explore your emotions to identify where self-healing and self-care is needed. This book is for you to improve your quality of life, the quality and scope of your healing work, and it is an opportunity to look and see what isn't working. Then, you can begin to work with your body and mind for continual improvement. You can bring the best version of yourself to the "healing field" that you create with each of your patients or clients.

Obviously, these recommendations are not a replacement for your unique healing method. Hopefully the information in this book will give you a fresh perspective and maybe some new thoughts on the complexity of the body-mind and healing. They are meant to assist and aid you in being an active part of your own healing, bringing awareness for more balance, peace, and harmony.

Enhance your health, enhance your life, and face your challenges in a new way.

- Whether you believe in all of this woo-woo stuff or not, it won't hurt you to explore the possible benefits to your health and your life.

- Science has proven for years that using the power of our minds, emotions and bodies to improve our lives, works. Get over your limited thinking.

- Throughout this book, challenge your subconscious beliefs (the ones you didn't choose that you absorbed from the environment you grew up in). Begin to set your own conscious beliefs by crafting your personal approach to an open-minded perspective.

- Realize that this process of energy integration is a missing part of most people's Health Code.

Chapter 1
Eyes Opened

We must be willing to get rid of the life we've planned so as to have the life that's waiting for us.

Joseph Campbell

I had been interested in why repetitive injuries happened to some of my patients. Each day, patients came and went in their usual manner, telling me about their aches, pains, and physical challenges. I had seen patterns within each patient's symptoms and between similar characteristics among groups of patients. I had seen in them a relationship with the events of a car accident trauma and what was happening in their minds at the same time.

For example, I would treat a patient's injuries after an auto accident where he had been sitting at a stop light while it was raining; there was a crash of thunder, screeching of tires, then the impact of a rear-end collision. The patient would heal from his injuries and we would release him from care. Then a few months later, he returned to my office with the same or similar physical symptoms. On questioning, I discovered that although he had been sitting again at a stoplight on a rainy night and there was a crash of thunder with a screech of tires, there had been no collision. The next morning, all the original whiplash symptoms of neck and upper back pain, stiffness, and headache had returned. I was curious how the body remembered the physical trauma by merely recreating the sights, sounds, and feelings of the original accident.

Cases like this piqued my interest in how the mind and body experience all of the sensations of trauma. I was fascinated by how the body remembers these sensations and links them with pain. I have helped patients by working our way through all of their symptoms and exploring the emotions they had at the time of an accident.

With the use of visualization and breathing processes, we were able to unlock the blocked emotional energy in the tissues. These processes not only released the emotions associated with the trauma, but also released the cycle of pain and symptoms as well. As I observed this in patient after patient, I began to wonder if this body-mind collaboration occurred in other experiences throughout our lives.

My mind realized one day with "Mary" (not her real name, and all examples have the name changed) that body-mind synergy truly does exist. In the midst of my flow of patients, she came complaining of a severe migraine. She was a new patient having her first visit and it looked like Mary would not tolerate a complete physical exam. Her headache was so severe that she could hardly stand up or walk straight without assistance. Turning or moving her head was a disaster. She wore dark sunglasses and a hooded sweatshirt to block any light from her eyes. My staff moved her to the darkest room in the clinic and had her recline on a treatment table.

I knew manual manipulation of her spine was out of the question. Soft tissue muscle work and massage would be impossible because of her sensitivity to touch. My only hope, other than sending her to the hospital for painkillers, was to work with her body-to-mind communication in order to learn what was triggering this migraine episode. I asked her if she wanted to go to the hospital. She resoundingly replied, "No! That's why I came here!" I then asked her if she was open to exploring the emotional connection to her migraine, since anything I could do physically would probably just increase her discomfort. She pleaded, "Anything. Just help me."

I started by using deep breathing and allowing Mary to become more deeply aware of her body. I helped her open her body-mind communication through a visualization process that helped her link her pain to the unresolved trauma stored in her body. Through this process we discovered that she was suppressing an incredibly charged emotional event she had experienced with her boss earlier that day. This led us to a memory of her earlier childhood experience of her father yelling at her. She was able to feel and experience the fear mixed with confusion she had when she was a child. Her confusion we found was from being wakened in the night to the sound of her father and mother screaming at each other, where they would often be throwing things. She remembered witnessing the physical abuse of her mother at these times as well.

These memories were suppressed when she was a child. She was unable to find an outlet for the build-up of this emotional energy in her body. She had no way to allow this deep fear along with the feelings of helplessness and hopelessness to be expressed. Dr. Peter Levine speaks to this phenomenon in his book, In an Unspoken Voice, when he poses the question asking what is a therapist to do when presented with a human being who is hurt and beaten down by past trauma? Dr. Levine states we should help people listen to the unspoken voice of their own bodies. We can enable them to feel their "survival emotions" of rage and terror without being overwhelmed by these powerful states. Trauma, as Levine writes, does not reside in the external event that induces physical or emotional pain. It resides in our becoming stuck in our primitive responses to painful events. Trauma is caused when we are unable to release blocked energies, to fully move through the physical/emotional reactions to hurtful experiences. Trauma is not what happens to us, but what we hold inside until we are in the presence of someone who can assist us in releasing our emotions and associated physiology. Someone who can be an empathetic witness to their experience.

The salvation and solution, then, is to be found in the body. "Most people," Levine notes, "think of trauma as a mental problem, even as a brain disorder." But we now know that trauma is something that also happens in the body. In fact, he shows it happens first and foremost in the body. The mental states associated with trauma are important, but they are secondary. The body initiates, his work notes, and the mind follows.

I have learned that the therapist/healer needs to be able to recognize the psychoemotional and physical signs of trauma in clients. He or she must learn to hear the "unspoken voice" of the body so that clients can safely learn to be body aware. Like my patient Mary, we know that potential traumatic situations are ones that induce states of high physiological arousal. However, without the freedom for the affected person to express and get past these states, their body creates symptoms (migraine in Mary's case) to help the person become aware of their stuck or frozen unexpressed emotional energy. In simpler language, danger without the possibility of fight or flight only leaves the "freeze" state of trauma. Afterward, the client is left without the opportunity to "shake it off," as a wild animal would following a frightful encounter with a predator. This is what ethologists call tonic immobility. Tonic immobility is the paralysis and physical/ emotional shutdown that characterizes the universal experience of helplessness in the face of perceived mortal danger. If this experience of helplessness is not "shaken off", then this deeper unresolved trauma comes to dominate the person's life. It will dominate how his or her body functions. We are literally frozen by our pain or "scared stiff."

In human beings, unlike in animals, the state of temporary freezing becomes a long-term trait. The survivor, Levine illustrates, may remain "stuck in a kind of limbo, not fully reengaging in life". In future circumstances, a triggering incident where others may sense no more than a mild threat, the traumatized person experiences threat, dread, and mental/physical listlessness, even often, physical pain. They experience a kind of paralysis of body and will. Shame, depression, and self-loathing follow in the wake of such imposed helplessness. In the case with Mary, she was feeling all of these things and they were creating a migraine headache as a symptom.

In an effort to be that empathetic witness for Mary, I continued to follow the path of her body and mind as they worked together and made the linkages of her specific limiting beliefs and suppressed emotions connected with this migraine. Through my evaluation of her physical body, it was evident that she had neck, mid-back, and jaw tension. This tension in the fascia or soft tissue structures reduces blood flow to the area. It also causes an over-stimulation of the nerves, a tightening of the fascia throughout the body and brain and therefore a reduction of oxygen to tissues, causing pain.

She was in a safe space to be guided through breathing and some uncontrolled movement of her body. This body movement was her body releasing the old trauma. She would shake, vibrate, and toss gently back and forth. This release of old trauma is genetically part of our animal nature. It is how we appropriately let the body unwind or release the energy from our muscles and central nervous system—we literally "shake it off". We instinctively discharge the traumatic energy in a positive way.

As we ended our session she sat upright. She removed her shaded glasses. She looked around and said, "Wow, that was interesting." I agreed. Her migraine went away while she was in the office and she continued to improve with time. For the eight years that I continued to follow her case, her migraine headaches did not return. Amazing? The body and mind together make a remarkable system of healing that continues to teach and inspire me.

I was stunned and in awe of the body's ability to heal in such a precise and eloquent way. The end result of this healing was an increase in Mary's awareness of the cause of her migraines and the relief of the symptoms. This was the beginning of my study, research, and continual quest to better understand this body-mind innate and instinctual communication.

This book reviews how in most instances our body is giving us signals, often represented in our bodies as symptoms, pain or disease. John E. Sarno, MD, discusses in his book The Divided Mind

> . . . the altered physiology [in what he terms TMS, Tension Myositis Syndrome] appears to be a mild, localized reduction in blood flow to a small region or specific body structure, such as a spinal nerve, resulting in a state of mild oxygen deprivation. The result is pain, the primary symptom. The tissues that may be targeted by the brain include the muscles of the neck, shoulders, back or buttocks, any spinal or peripheral nerve and any tendon. As a consequence,

symptoms may occur virtually anywhere in the body. The nature of the pain varies depending on the tissues involved: muscle, nerve or tendon. In addition to pain, nerve involvement brings with it the possibility of feelings of numbness and tingling and/or actual muscle weakness. The fact that patients recover rapidly when they are appropriately treated suggests that the tissues involved—nerve tissue being the most sensitive—are not in any way damaged but only rendered temporarily dysfunctional.

As a Chiropractor, I know how every cell, tissue, and organ in the body can respond to these temporary dysfunctions that Dr. Sarno writes about. I have charted, with the help of others, how specific emotions tend to relate through the nervous system to all areas of the body and organ systems.

When I refer to the association between organs and parts of the body with links to specific possible emotions in this book, I mean something significant that is "hidden" or "whispering", a deeper issue wanting attention for resolution. Your body has the ability to show you through these symptoms or whispers where you are holding unresolved emotional events or traumas. The messages aren't all negative—these old unresolved echoes can assist us in our personal growth. They can be the missing piece to our complete healing. Through becoming body-aware we can release these repressed emotions, which will release patterns that keep us stuck in unhappy relationships, unfulfilling careers, and in a limiting life. In the process, we can identify and rewrite those limiting life stories that inhibit us from the lives we want to live. In addition, we experience a healthier body along with a peaceful mental and emotional path in our lives. When we listen to the whispers, we can begin to construct an insightful story that will unveil for us where we are out of balance in our lives. If we can utilize these stories to take action, we can heal our bodies (symptoms), and also improve and enhance the quality of our lives.

Working through these stories and imbalances with my clients opened the door for me to apply this same healing in my own life. Once I decided to look deeply into what was working and not working within myself, I experienced many and numerous epiphanies into what I needed for personal responsibility in my journey through cancer. There are too many to discuss here, but one thing I discovered was that writing this book was a must. Know that all of the recommendations in this book are methods I still use personally and with clients every day in my practice. The concepts and ideas are still valid today and are backed by current scientific research.

Part of my healing on this journey has been to tap into that suppressed creative aspect of myself and share it for others to enjoy, from which they may learn, and hopefully use to heal. The research on pain and discomfort is overflowing with information about body-mind and reciprocal influences facilitating our healing. Research shows how brain wave changes during meditation, deep breathing, and body awareness and how they collaborate to allow more effective self-care. All of this research helps make the link between the body and our stored unexpressed emotions. In chiropractic therapies, my friend and colleague, Dr. Scott Walker, developed the Neuro-Emotional Technique that helps us understand how the study of chiropractic, body physiology, acupuncture meridians, and the chakra systems link with the brain to create neuroemotional complexes.

In complementary fashion, Dr. Ida Rolf conducted research to inform us of how emotions and traumatic experiences get stuck in the fascia of the body and in our soft tissues. Soft tissues are our muscles, ligaments, tendons, and organs systems. Similarly, regarding emotions and soft tissues, John E. Sarno, MD, states:

> The type of symptom and its location in the body is not important, the cause is to be found in the unconscious regions of the mind, and its purpose is to deliberately distract the conscious mind. On occasion, the choice of symptom location may even contribute to the diversion process, for example, a man who experiences the acute onset of pain in the arm while swinging a tennis racket will naturally assume that it was something about the swing that hurt his arm. The reality is that his brain has decided that the time is

ripe for a physical diversion and chooses that moment to initiate the pain, because the person will assume that it stems from an injury, not a brain-generated physical condition that generated the pain. If this seems bizarre, diabolical, or self-destructive, it is in reality a protective maneuver. My colleagues and I have observed it in thousands of patients.

As Sarno says, these "physical diversions" are where we can use our pains, strains, and symptoms to look deeper at the insightful stories our body and mind are revealing to us. Then, in seeing where we are stuck, we can have access to actions that will free us. Often these stuck patterns are held in place by our inability to completely process the emotions at the time of the experience. The mind stores these unprocessed emotions in our body until the right combination of resources are available to process them appropriately or to heal them. Until these unprocessed emotions are healed, they will be expressed throughout our lives subconsciously (meaning we may not be aware) in the form of pain, disease processes, or repetitive destructive behavior patterns. These limiting beliefs can drive our behaviors, attitudes, perceptions, and even the expression of our genes.

Once incorporated into our soft tissues through energy pathways or simply neurological pathways, the limiting beliefs and unresolved emotions create all kinds of havoc. These emotions create chronic pain syndromes, dysfunction of a joint, or improper enzyme activity in an organ system. It is proven that environmental signaling to the genes through our behaviors, attitudes, perceptions, and beliefs can activate or suppress gene expression. Cellular biologist Bruce Lipton, PhD, shares that through the science of epigenetics we have learned that our lives are determined not by our genes themselves, but by our genes' responses to the environmental signals that operate in our lives. Some of the strongest environmental signals are internally generated by our emotional responses, beliefs, attitudes, behaviors and perceptions. In simple terms, our wellness and quality of our life is based upon how we perceive and respond to the challenges in our lives. The activity of our genes is constantly being modified in response to life experiences (our perceptions).

Emotional and mental states affect our bodies. The effects can provide an understanding of what is happening in our body-mind communication. This book will provide some tools that will allow you as a healer to be more aware of the mental/ emotional components. It can guide your conversation with your client to find the meaning behind presenting symptoms or circumstances that may be creating pain in their body, or aid them to recognize destructive behaviors or patterns in their life.

Our bodies give us insights into what is happening in our mental, emotional, and physical environment. When our lives are out of balance, our bodies are out of balance. With the imbalance, we experience pain or discomfort. If we pay attention to these warning signs or "insights" we can understand the lesson, change our behavior or perspective, and then move forward on our path. Typically, over time we have developed ways to suppress or numb rather than deal with the underlying emotional trauma, shame, anxiety, or self-loathing. Sometimes we default to taking medication, alcohol, or other substances to block the feelings rather than addressing it—this is why the pain persists. As a healer this is fertile soil to create personal growth and healing for your patients.

Recently, I experienced this myself. I was rolling along in my life, eating well, managing my mind as well as emotions, and exercising every day. I had the belief that I was maintaining a lifestyle that would prevent disease. Then, I was diagnosed with aggressive, large B Cell Non-Hodgkin's Lymphoma. My oncologist said I was about two weeks from dying by the time I was diagnosed, and my PET scan showed over 150 active lymph node tumors throughout my chest cavity, abdomen, and pelvis. I was in the hospital for five days beginning my treatment and being managed closely for complications. During those five days I spent many hours reflecting on my life. I explored the emotional/mental stresses and upsets as well as the life stories that may have contributed to my condition. Since diet, exercise, and having a good mindset had not prevented my cancer, then there must have been some stories, perceptions, attitudes, beliefs or emotions that created an environment favorable to generating cancer in my body. As Dr. Lipton might say, my environmental signals were creating a disease message to my gene expression. Yes, there were toxic environmental factors that have known links to my and other types of cancers. All cancers are unfortunate and random events in too many peoples' lives. But I knew that if I was going to thrive rather than just survive, I had to control how I was going to respond to my treatment and recovery. So, exploring and healing my emotions, thoughts, and beliefs was imperative. Then, creating a more empowering mindset was how I was going to thrive.

I reminded myself of a teaching by Ryan Holiday in the podcast and website, The Daily Stoic, where Epictetus tells the story of Agrippinus, who, during Nero's reign, was suddenly and unexpectedly given some awful news. The awful news was that he was exiled, effective immediately. Agrippinus's response was likewise swift. "Very well, we shall take our lunch in Aricia," (a city nearby and outside the city from which he was exiled). He was determined to move forward without bemoaning or weeping about it. The time to change and get on with the task at hand had arrived. We learn from this story to shrug off the emotional weight of even the worst news, to focus on what we can control and release that which we cannot. If you practice, if you rehearse, if you strengthen yourself for the fact that life inevitably will deliver these moments to us—being exiled, getting fired, hearing that your computer just deleted a year of hard work, getting a bad diagnosis—you can take action on what you can control. Knowing that none of that is fun, that it may often feel unfair you could let it crush you and you could fall on your knees and ask, "Why me?" Instead, you should decide you are going to find a way to thrive, not just survive.

When I looked into the emotional component of Lymphoma, I made some discoveries: my Lymphoma was associated with unprocessed feelings of resentment and resignation; Lymphoma relates to feelings of running on empty with insufficient resources to replenish your energy; it also relates to feelings of "what is the use?", with an abiding anger about a situation. I felt like I had to suffer silently and to stuff my sorrow. As I learned more, I also realized that I had a subconscious belief that I always come up "a day late and a dollar short" as a function of how the world works. I had the perception that I didn't have the right to request or require, much less complain about my situation. I was not dealing with these beliefs, perceptions, and attitudes because I had a poorly developed ability to nurture myself. I had been feeling all of these emotions on a subconscious level and, therefore, storing them in my lymphatic system. I had been feeling these emotions for quite some time, especially over the previous three years.

I also realized that about four years prior I had made a soul commitment to myself that I needed to change the nature of my practice. You see, I had left practice for a year in order to reorganize my approach to healing. My wife and I moved to Panama and tried our hands at retirement. We both had a number of realizations during that year, not the least of which for me was that I had 35 years of experience working with clients in their healing processes. Here I was, retired, and my 35 years of experience were just going to go to waste. I knew during that year away from my healing practice that I wanted to return to work. I wanted to teach patients self-healing, self-care education, and help them understand their potential for healing at a deeper level. I knew I wanted to share my clinical experiences with other healers. I knew there was more to share and always more to learn from others. I made a soul agreement—you know, one of those moments when you commit to doing something by saying, "I will not be deterred or allow myself to drift off this path, this commitment, it is that important to me."

We left Panama and I re-entered practice. As deep-seated behaviors tend to work, I found myself working my practice in my old, comfortable way as I always had. I had a nagging inner desire to change my practice, from one of surface level healing to working more deeply with the root cause of patients' pain and their life imbalances. I want to share self-healing and self-care strategies using the principles in this book. Yet three years later, I was immobilized to create that change. I felt that the "breaking" of my soul agreement with myself was coming back to make me face the music, so to speak, through this challenge of cancer. I knew I needed to help clients find what was driving their pain by identifying their deeper mental and emotional traumas. I wanted to help them bring their limiting life stories to light so they could see how their emotions and beliefs were affecting their overall behavior. In the process, the outcome of my work would be to help them find fulfillment in their own lives.

What created the healing for me was not only the medical treatment I was receiving, but also my exploration into my own emotional/mental and spiritual blocks. I had been ignoring these blocks for a long time, but more so over the last three to four years. It was during my cancer treatment that I committed to changing my approach to my work and began to heal my own body and mind. The result was astonishing, and it continues to be an incredible journey.

This book is meant to inform and educate about the ways you can empower yourself to heal and be the best version of yourself in the world. With that empowerment, you then can bring that best version to your healing practice. It is about taking back your responsibility, your power for self-healing. Then, being a powerful healing force in others' lives. Use the information to learn emotional insights commonly associated with many of the areas of the body. Throughout the book, I explain my own experience of healing and many of the methods I use with clients. I hope to put you on the path of self-healing and self-care that will inspire you to create the life you want. That will inspire you to use what you learn from your own experience to assist others in their own healing. It will be transformative to you and to your clients.

Awareness Keys

- Our amazing body-mind remembers every detail of our experiences. Any element of that original memory can trigger a physiological cascade of symptoms in your body. You can use these experiences to extinguish the symptoms and to learn and grow from these triggers.

- Sometimes the best thing we can do to heal is to breathe, release the associated emotions, and let our bodies "shake it off". Let your body move and unwind at the physical level.

- Realize that there is an abundant source of energy in the Universe. Call it God, Mother Nature, Source, Universal Intelligence or whatever. It is flowing through you and is the generator of your power to heal.

- You may have challenges show up for you in various ways once you decide to heal, to grow, and to have the life you want. This is not the time to throw in the towel and quit. It is the time to claim your power and use the tools to be a better version of yourself.

- As you will see later in this book, years of study and compilation of data give us a roadmap as to what we might want to explore emotionally. Exploring the emotional elements of injury to a body part or a less than healthy organ system can be the end of pain. Emotional and mental states affect our bodies. The feelings in our bodies then become triggers to the way our minds choose to think. This is the definition of addiction. We become addicted to our emotions.

- Our genes either do or don't express themselves based on the environmental stimuli they are subjected to. In other words, how you think, feel and behave influences how your genes act. You are creating an environment of life enhancement or disease production.

- No matter what your current challenge: health, life sucks, career is not something you love, don't let it crush you. Make the changes in your mind, emotions, and behaviors to thrive.

- This book gives you a roadmap to explore playing a responsible part in your own healing and self-care. The point is you must take the action to honor yourself and remember that you are the most valuable asset in the entire Universe.

Chapter 2
Bottom-Up Thinking

What lies behind us and what lies before us are tiny matters compared to what lies within us.

Ralph Waldo Emerson

As a society we don't talk much about emotions. Conversations tend to focus more on what we are doing or what we are thinking. Most of the time we find it less awkward and easier to start a sentence with "I think" instead of "I feel." Many of us were never educated about feelings. There are segments of the community who weren't fortunate enough to grow up surrounded by emotionally superb role models and, so, likely missed out on important emotional concepts. Most people, if they haven't had the clinical experiences I have in practice, might think that emotions are just an aspect of the brain and how it functions. This is understandable, since the history of medicine was based on the Cartesian Theory (the philosophical and scientific system of René Descartes and other seventeenth century thinkers). The Cartesians viewed the mind as being entirely separate from the physical body. The mind (including emotions and feelings) is the domain of the "shrinks" and the body is the domain of medicine. It's important to recognize that much of medicine today still operates under the Cartesian Theory. This means you and your clients have been raised in a culture that doesn't always recognize that the mind and body are actually one system of interconnected thoughts, emotions, feelings, and physical responses.

Current neuroscience teaches us a significant amount about emotion and its relationship to our body. The Cartesian top-down model, where the "higher" brain controls the "lower" functions of the body (i.e. the digestive system), has been turned upside down by neuropathologist Dr. Paul Ivan Yakovlev of the Harvard School of Medicine. It was Dr. Yakovlev's contention that our more complex and specialized parts of the thinking brain are an evolutionary refinement, ultimately derived from emotional and visceral functions including ingestion, digestion, and elimination. In other words, the brain is a gadget evolved by the stomach to serve the purpose of securing food. Likewise, the more typical medical model, Cartesian top-down theory states that the stomach is a device invented by the brain to provide it with the energy and raw materials it needs to function and stay alive. Both concepts are equally true and we know from science that this is how organisms function. Brain (mind) to organs (body) and organs (body) to brain (mind). This difference in perspective is not just wordplay. The whole concept that the organ systems of the body generate the development of the thinking brain implies an entirely different worldview. It entirely alters the outlook on how you and your bodywork can impact your ability to heal.

This is really important to understand when we begin to look at how emotions are related to body parts and organ systems (known as viscera). Yakovlev believed that brain development is a function of the primitive needs of the organs. What this means is that the more primitive brain centers gave rise to the higher levels of brain function—the hypothalamus, limbic system, and the cortex. The primitive brain centers control and takes direction from the organ systems of the body. We actually feel and think with our guts. The digestive process, as an example, is initially experienced as a physical sensation (hunger), then as an emotional feeling (hunger as motivation or aggression) that drives our thinking brain to go get food. This is also captured in our cultural language when we refer to or assimilate new thoughts, perceptions or concepts into our thinking. For example, we may say that we have a hunger for knowledge or that we need to digest a concept or idea. What we would call our higher thought process might indeed be a servant rather than a master. This is a bottom-up perspective instead of the typical top-down perspective. This bottom-up perspective is valuable in our emotional healing. It allows us to use our body symptoms to explore our thinking minds and our emotional bodies.

Neuroscience shows us in brain dissection that the very front of the brain, the prefrontal cortex, responsible for the most complex functions of human behavior, personality expression and decision making, curves anatomically all the way around the cranium. It makes a near U-turn and snuggles against the primitive brain stem and the limbic system. The limbic system is considered the emotional center of our brain. Neuroscience teaches that generally when two parts of the brain are in anatomical closeness, it is because they are meant to function together. This makes it even more likely that the electrochemical signals will be reliably shared between those adjacent parts. If the philosopher Descartes had the information about the brain that we do today, he might have been utterly awestruck at such an intimate relationship between the most primitive and most refined portions of the brain.

As next-door neighbors, brain stem, emotional brain, and thinking brain must find a common language with which to communicate. That common language is "subtle energy". The subtle energy of the primitive brain automatically controls heart rate, breathing, digesting foods, and sleep. Our thinking brain interprets higher functions like touch, vision, hearing, speech, and learning. Remarkably, the primitive and thinking parts of the brain must cohabitate and communicate with our emotional brain (limbic system) that controls the basic emotions (anger, fear, pleasure) and drives (hunger, sex, dominance, care of offspring). All three parts of the brain must communicate in a congruent and coherent harmony with the body. The primitive brain's rhythmic need to automatically control heart rate, breathing, digestion and sleep. The limbic system's need for emotional connection and processing of emotions. The thinking brain's function of perceiving, planning, judgment, initiation, impulse control, and social and sexual behavior converge where all of these parts meet. This creates the synchrony of creating and living our life story. It determines whether our life story is empowering or not. It shapes how we integrate all of the energy aspects of our body with the life stories we live and tell ourselves and how this influences our health and wellbeing.

This is the meat and potatoes of how emotional healing works. The combination of the three parts of our brain interacting with the ancient Chinese meridian systems, the chakra systems, our nervous system, and our bodies all function together for our ultimate healing. These systems communicate in various ways through subtle energies. For example, current practices in Western medicine measure different types of subtle energy in the human body by using diagnostic procedures including ones you are familiar with; including sonograms, x-rays, MRIs (magnetic resonant imaging), electrocardiograms, and electroencephalograms to name a few. Quantum physics teaches us that there is no difference between energy and matter. All systems in the human being—from the atomic to the molecular level—are expressing subtle energy and are currently in motion creating resonance. This is how subtle energy directs and maintains health and wellness in the human being. While modern medicine focuses primarily on physiology, the human organism has many aspects that are not physical. All of the body systems are really channels for energy communication. The methods used in this book are accessing these same energy channels and subtle energy fields to treat energetic imbalances in the Human Energy Field (HEF) bringing the body's systems back to homeostasis. It is known that disturbances in the coherence of the energy patterns of the HEF are indications of disease and aging. When these energy patterns are brought back into coherent energy alignment through the methods in this book and other energy medicine treatments, the disturbed energy patterns return to their original coherent, harmonic, resonant states (homeostasis).

Resonance

The communication between invisible resonance and physical manifestation on a conscious level is imperceptible and yet is an incredibly powerful force in our lives. This subtle energy is operating, in fact whispering, to all aspects of our being on a subconscious level. The interplay between systems in and around the body as well as mind is accomplished by subtle energy interactions. Here is where invisible vibrations wait to take physical form. This subtle energy phenomenon is the basis for all that we are: thoughts, emotions, cells, organs and systems, and how they interact in addition to relate to each other. The amazing part of this is that our nervous system, fascial matrix, cell receptors, and genes are capable of sensing these whispering vibrations of subtle energy. All of these complex coordinated systems with their extraordinary sensitivity and feedback loops between the body and the brain are what is considered our body-mind.

When you take the world in through your senses, it is actually subtle energy, resonant frequency, which is coming into your being. The form itself does not come into your mind and body; the form stays outside, and we actually resonate with the experience. But it is processed by your senses into energy patterns that your body-mind receives and experiences. We know resonance when we experience it. When we resonate with an experience, we feel connected to the source of that experience. We may say, "I feel connected, I feel more like myself." If feels this way whether it comes from the perfect words of a speech or when a rock band plays at a concert. At a concert, the harmonies of the music resonate with the human energy field (soul) through hearing and vibration to create a shared resonance experience in listeners. Those people at the concert are bonded together in a shared experience of vibration, frequency, and sensation that can connect thousands into one resonant, cohesive body. Scientists explain the sensory process like this: Your eyes are not really windows through which you look onto the world. Your eyes are cameras that pick up electronic images of the world and send these electronic waves of energy into your brain where it is converted to the image. Sound vibrations and energy waves are converted in the brain into audible patterns that then become interpretations of the world around us.

This is true of all of your senses. Our senses take in the world, convert the images, light, sound, electricity, or magnetism into information, transmit the data through the chakra and central nervous systems, and then the impressions get written in your mind. Your senses are indeed energy data-sensing mechanisms. But if the energy patterns coming into your body-mind are interpreted as an energy pattern disturbance, then you will resist them and not allow them to pass through you. When this happens, it creates disharmony in the entire energy system of the body. When there is disharmony in the energy patterns, then the body and mind aren't sure what to do with these disturbances. Without letting them pass through you or being able to resolve the disturbance, the body then stores the disturbance until the time that it can resolve them or return to homeostasis, a return to resonance.

We all experience resonance as a feeling, but in fact resonance follows the laws of physics and the observations and principles of science. When you tune your radio to 106.3, the receiver is resonating with the signal being sent out by the antenna that is transmitting at 106.3. Only that station is received at that site on the dial. The receiver and transmitter are resonating at the same frequency. Without resonance, all of our modern digital communication systems would not exist. My friend and colleague, Dr. Carol McMakin explains it this way: "When you open your car door with a key, it changes the lock from closed to open mechanically. When you use the key fob, it opens the door with a signal that connects with only your car door lock, not any of the others in the parking lot. It can resonate with the front door, or trunk, or passenger doors. The locks are tuned to respond to the signal from that key fob and no other. That is resonance."

An important thing to remember about all of this energy and frequency talk is that, for most of us, it doesn't seem real. If we can't perceive the energy, then we must be just making it up. The problem with this way of thinking is we are operating with a nervous system and sensory system in our bodies that only have the capacity to experience a certain range of frequencies. There are many different frequencies of light that are in our world; however, our eyes only interpret a small fraction of those frequencies. The world of sound frequencies is vast and, for humans, mostly imperceptible. Dogs have a broader ability to hear frequencies which is why they can perceive the seemingly "silent" dog whistle. Our auditory sensory system only has the capacity to experience a small range of these frequencies. But, even though we can't hear, see, or feel radio frequencies, we can still perceive them. I bring this to mind here so that as we proceed in this book you remember that just because the limited range of your sensory system doesn't perceive it, it doesn't mean that your nervous system with its much larger range of perception doesn't experience it.

To understand this better, imagine that nothing got blocked or stored inside of you; what if everything passed right through you without creating a disturbance? Think about walking down the sidewalk passing objects. While you are walking, you see buildings, trees, people, cars—none of these make lasting impressions on you. It is just a fleeting glimpse that allows you to see them, but they don't "stick" with you because as quickly as they are made, they are released. When you have no personal attachment with things, they process freely through bio-emotional gateways, chakras, and the nervous system.

This is how the overall system of perception is meant to work. It is meant to see things, experience them, and then let them pass through you so you are fully present in the next moment. When this system of perception is in a fully operative state, you are fine and the system operates well, experience after experience. They are passing into you, awakening you, stimulating you, and allowing you to have a life of abundant experiences. Experiences are occurring moment after moment, creating a profound effect on you, allowing you to learn and grow. Your energy centers and mind are expanding; you are being touched at a very deep level. What it means to live life is to experience the moment that is passing through you and then experience the next moment and then the next.

But this is not what happens in most of us. Instead, it is more like you are riding with a friend in a car down the street, seeing the same things as you did on the walk where the visuals create no disturbance, but then something comes along that doesn't pass through. Maybe it's seeing two people at a table near the front window of a café. The one person looks just like a friend with whom you had a disagreement. Well, at least it sure looked like your friend. But, you try to think, it probably was just another person just like all of the others whom you have noticed along the street, or was it? No, it wasn't just like all the other people to you. And your energy shifts.

Look carefully at what actually happened. Surely for the camera of the eye there was no difference between that person in the café window and the others that you noticed as you passed along the street. There is light bouncing off of objects passing through your retina and making a visual impression on your mind. So at the physical level, nothing different is happening. At the mental level, the impression on your mind didn't make it through. When the next moment comes, you no longer notice the buildings, the people moving about, or the rest of the scenes. You're not seeing the rest of the people moving around, either; your heart and mind are fixated on that one person even though the visual experience is gone.

Now you've got a disturbance in the flow of your energy. There is a blockage, an event that got stuck. All the subsequent experiences that are trying to pass through you are stunted because something inside has happened that has left this past experience unfinished. What has happened to the image of the person in a café if it doesn't just fade away into deep memory like everything else? At some point, you will have to stop focusing on it in order to deal with something else. What you don't realize is your entire experience of life is about to change because of what didn't flow flawlessly through your bio-emotional gateways, chakras, and nervous systems. Life must now compete with this blocked event for your attention and get around that impression.

When you have a disturbance, you probably already know that your tendency is to think about it constantly. This is in an attempt to find a way to process it through your body-mind. You didn't need to process the trees, but you need to process this because you resisted. It got stuck. Now you have disharmony in your rhythm. Then you notice new thoughts start to arise and take your attention. These new thoughts take your attention away from the current moment. Well maybe it wasn't her, of course it wasn't her, how could that possibly have been her? Thought after thought repeats incessantly inside of your mind. This inner noise is your attempt to process the blocked energy and get it out of the way. Long term, the energy patterns that can't make it through you get pushed out of the forefront of the mind and held in the body and the human energy field (HEF) until you are prepared to release them. They don't just disappear.

When you are unable to allow life's events to pass through you, they stay inside and can throw your systems off rhythm. These patterns may be held inside you for a very long time. These energy patterns hold tremendous detail about the events associated with them, and their effects are real. The body and mind expend a tremendous amount of energy holding onto this stuck energy. As you willfully struggle to keep these events from passing through your consciousness, several things occur. The energy first tries to release by manifesting through the mind. This is why the mind becomes so active. When the energy can't make it through the mind because there is conflict with other thoughts and mental concepts, it then tries to release through the body and the energy centers (called gateways). This is what creates painful signs and symptoms—emotional energy that may start or add to a disease process within the body. When you resist releasing energy in the moment, it gets packed up and forced in deep storage within the gateways, chakras, body parts, or organ systems.

My friend Dr. Carol McMakin states it this way: when there are two tuned violins in the same room and you bow the G string on one of them, the G string on the other violin will begin to vibrate on the other side of the room. The vibrations from the first string travel through the air and resonate with only the other G string. No other thing will vibrate except the one that is tuned to match G. That is resonance. If there is a weight or a finger on the G string, it won't vibrate in response to the other G string. The obstruction stops the vibration that should happen when the matching G string is bowed. That's interference. When you remove the interference and allow the string to respond to its essential frequency, it will hum in response to the G string from across the room. Resonance happens when there is no interference between the source and the receiver. If there is a building in between your key fob and your car, the door won't open because of the interference. When you come into the line of sight with your car, the interference is removed and the door lock will open. Resonance happens when the interference is removed.

In his book, The Untethered Soul, Michael Singer tells us that in the yogic tradition unfinished stored energy patterns are called samskaras, a Sanskrit word meaning "impression". In the yogic traditions, an unfinished energy impression is considered one of the most important influences affecting your life. A samskara is a blockage, an interference, an impression from your past, operating as an unfinished energy pattern that ends up ruining your life. Samskara is a cycle of stored past energy patterns in a state of relative equilibrium, but that's not the problem per se. What causes the issue is your resistance to experiencing these patterns, which causes these energy patterns to continue spinning. There is no other place for them to go. You won't let them leave. This packet of cycling energy has to be stored, and it sits in your energetic heart center or other energetic organ systems in your body. All the samskaras you have collected over your life are stored in these places and act like an infection of what is intended to be pure open energetic space.

Now, take a moment and go back to the event of seeing what looked like your friend with whom you recently argued in that café window. Once the disturbed energy patterns are packaged and stored in your energetic bio-emotional centers, they may feel to you like they are basically inactive. It may feel that you have handled the situation and that you have no more issues with that experience. You may not even mention the event to your friend with you in the car because it might make you seem distracted from your time together and the enjoyment you were having until that particular moment. So you don't talk about it, process it, or deal with it in any way. You didn't know what to do with this impression, so you resisted the energy flowing through you. It got stored in the body where you assumed it could fall into the background and not be bothersome. Well, it may seem like it is done, over, and gone. It really isn't. This interference blocks your resonance.

Everything that doesn't make it through you from the time you were a baby all the way up to this moment is still inside of your energy field. Take the example of my patient, Mary, who was being yelled at by her boss. Her samskaras from many years ago (that she witnessed as a child about her mother and father fighting, and the impressions of physical or emotional abuse) that had been all stuffed away inside her were triggered. They got activated. It is these impressions, these samskaras that, once activated for Mary, generated her migraine. For all of us, samskaras block the free flow of consciousness in our lives and upset our natural rhythm.

We all have these impressions and they amazingly store all of the energy of the original event in complete detail. These impressions include all of the emotions and thoughts you experienced at the time of the event as well as that event's energy pattern and nature. You, like in Mary's case, have years later moved on from the past event, but have a sensory experience (see something, hear a noise, taste a distant spice, feel a cold gust of wind, smell a distinctive scent that is associated with that past samskara) that activates that old energy. Granted, there are sensory reminders that trigger pleasant and happy memories, but we are focusing on the held old energy, not memories where the impression passed through you. When that old energy is triggered it releases and stimulates a physical response. For example, your heart actually starts beating faster; you start getting moody, irritated, and agitated.

All of these inner changes occurred because your energy balance was disturbed when you experienced one particular aspect of that old stuck memory or energy pattern. It is truly amazing how this process unfolds inside of you. A past event took place in your life for just a few moments, and a passing unrelated moment changes the energy pattern of your body-mind. As weird and hard to believe as this seems, it actually happens this way with everything that didn't make it through you. It is no wonder we are able to be overwhelmed pretty much at any time in our lives. As our bio-emotional gateways are constantly opening and closing, the energy that is stored there is real. It keeps interacting with the flow of current thoughts and events. The dynamics of these ongoing interactions with the stored energy cause the samskaras to become activated, sometimes years later. It doesn't have to be the exact same situation; anything could activate the energy of the samskara. Instantly you are experiencing the feeling that you had when the locked-up festering energy was trapped inside you.

What we are experiencing in these situations are unfinished mental and emotional energy patterns getting reactivated after being stored for long periods of time. Luckily, most of what washes over us from the world does not get blocked. Most things make it right through our gateways and for this we can be eternally grateful. The items that get stuck in our systems are the ones that cause disharmony.

"Sticking" occurs in two ways, though more frequently in society it's because there is some problem or painful event in our life. However, we can also get disharmony in our system from extraordinary experiences as well. When a wonderful experience occurs, it gets stuck because you become attached to it for good reasons. That incredible sunset when you were snuggled up with your love and sipping a great wine produces a desire to keep replaying that moment again and again. Clinging to this image, impression, or attachment causes positive samskaras that release positive energy.

Hence, two kinds of experiences can occur that block the mind, body, chakras, or other energy centers in the body. You are either trying to hide energies because they bother you or you are trying to keep them close because you like them. In both cases, you are not letting them pass through you. Unfortunately, you are wasting precious energy by blocking the flow by clinging and resisting to both good memory energy and not-so-hot events. There is an alternative—to enjoy life rather than pulling or pushing. If you can touch into these moments that show up for you in the form of stuck energy then use the methods in this book to release that energy, it may very well change your life.

The Path Less Taken

So, here is a metaphysical thought about how life could be. This will require you to open your mind a bit, but humor me. When we are born, we are given a birth certificate that has, among other things, our name, date of birth, time of birth, and location. That's it. Other than needing it in your life for a passport or some other legal document, this piece of paper is just that: a piece of paper that you seldom reference. There are some, myself included, who are open to being metaphysically oriented. This birth information can produce a natal chart run at the time of your entry on to the planet through various methods—astrology, I Ching, Cabala, Human Design, Ayurveda readings, or other information patterns. This is a roadmap of potentials and challenges that might present themselves in your life. This, in my thinking, is your true life story, which has many subtle influences and opportunities that may appear in your life at various times. If you are aware of these possibilities, potentials, or challenges that might present themselves at various times, you might be able to navigate your life with more insight and more forethought with less clinging or resisting. It is not necessarily your destiny, but it indicates possible energetic influences that might affect your decisions, your choices, and your path or direction that is best suited to your given gifts, talents, or abilities. Looking back, I wish I had been more aware of this information earlier in my life. I didn't get introduced to it until I was in my mid-30's. I personally think it is as useful as a personality profile, a strengths and weaknesses profile, or a behavioral test. It is much more inclusive of multiples of different subtle energy influences that are making an impact on our lives, our choices, our preferences, and our beliefs about who we truly are than you can imagine. The funny thing is we know these influences are there; we just tend to ignore them or at least we are not educated enough to use them effectively. If you are willing to let go of your resistance to experiences in your life and rewrite your current story, you will be moved to the depth of your being. We miss the fact that with our date and location, a resonance with the subtle energies of the Universe is set into motion that gives us a roadmap for our life story. With the use of Human Design, astrology of different forms, the enneagram, numerology, and I Ching, we have an insight into how the natural rhythm of our life story might unfold for us. We get insight into how we can resonate with our true purpose and path in life. As we become aware of and live our life story, we will discover conflict between the stories we been taught about ourselves. There is always a time in our lives, and the lives of our patients, when the cultural stories about how and who we "should" be collide with how and who we want to be. We will begin to identify these internal conflicting stories and ultimately heal them. Pain, discomfort, disease, stress, disharmony, and breakdown are all forms of incongruence of where the story we are currently living is in conflict with living the essence of our truly unique story. Becoming aware of where the interference to resonance exists, where we have been told or adopted life stories that are not truly ours, is where we block the flow of our own rhythm. If we could use the other energetic tools to find our stories and explore our natural gifts, talents, and rhythms, we would be able to live our lives from this harmonic place. I believe this is an aspect of the care of our clients and patients that many of us are missing as well. Imagine being able to help your clients who are struggling, in pain, stuck in a disempowering life story. Through the assistance of healers who are experts at many of these methods, we can help our patients find their own true life path. In this process we can assist them in healing the emotions that have been festering, we can clear the emotions that limit them from living fully, and we can help them develop powerful life enhancing emotions to step into the life story they want to build. Isn't this truly what our job is as doctors, therapists, coaches and healers? It might just be that easy. When the festering energetic impressions trigger you or you have the realization that you are living an incongruent life story, just smile. Show gratitude that this samskara that has been stored in your body now has the opportunity to make it through you and out of you. Just open and relax your heart, breathe, laugh, or do whatever creates freedom in your soul. Remind your clients to do the same when they are on your therapy bench and you see the stuck-ness. Of course, it is uncomfortable and even hurtful. It was stored with pain; it is going to release with discomfort and difficult choices. You have to decide if you want to live your unique story in the world. This is a profound way to consider living and fulfilling your destiny and your passion and purpose. This is a powerful and generous gift to your clients as well.

Harmony is returned by healing at the energy level. Once the appropriate resources are obtained by the body or mind in order to restore harmony, then healing can proceed on many levels. Bringing back harmony is like tuning a distorted-sounding instrument to allow the instrument to express the perfect vibration of sound for beautiful music. It also could be described as focusing or concentrating the normal broad scatter of light that we see in the visual spectrum into the concentrated, pinpoint light of a laser, which organizes regular light into coherent (harmonized) quantum vibrations. When light particles are in harmony, they can cut through steel! As you move through this book, you are going to learn to bring harmony to your life and the lives of your patients. With this harmony of energy and the practice of these new skills of healing, you can concentrate your energy like a laser. This focus will help you and your patients live a freer and increasingly flexible life.

Awareness Keys

- We don't talk much about emotions. In our culture we operate under the belief that if we only think things better they will be better. This is an exercise in futility.

- Our brains are amazing, but so are our bodies. It takes the full engagement of both body and mind to bring a significant shift in our consciousness and our ultimate healing—whether we are healing an injury, disease, or creating the life we truly want to live.

- Science tells us that our brain and body work together through a number of evolutionary systems including the chakra system, acupuncture system, central nervous system, hormonal system, just to mention a few.

- All of these vital systems communicate and operate through the exchange of subtle energy and vibrational frequencies.

- When our energy patterns or vibrational frequencies (resonance) are out of balance, we are open to injury, disease, or just bad decision making. Do you really make the best decisions when your life is in chaos or imbalance? Really?

- We all have stored samskaras that are less than positive energy patterns (memories if you want). Get over it. Face them and deal with them. Resolve them, push the extinction button and get on with creating a life worth living.

- Open your mind and your experiences in life to other ways of living and knowing yourself at a deeper level.

- Use available tools that have been around for your entire life. Let go of your thoughts that these tools are woo-woo, stupid, irrelevant or too out there.

- Explore astrology, natal charts, life path charts, Human Design analysis, and the enneagram to learn about possible subtle energy influences in your life. You never know, they may guide you to a life of fulfillment.

Chapter 3

Connections

"The atoms of our bodies are traceable to stars that manufactured them in their cores and exploded these enriched ingredients across our galaxy, billions of years ago. For this reason, we are biologically connected to every other living thing in the world. We are chemically connected to all molecules on Earth. And we are atomically connected to all atoms in the universe. We are not figuratively, but literally stardust."

— Neil deGrasse Tyson

We tend to see our bodies as fixed, solid, material objects, when in truth they are more like mountain streams that are constantly changing like flowing interactions of intelligence. The Greek philosopher, Heraclitus, stated, "You cannot step into the same river twice, for fresh waters are ever flowing in." We now know that the same principle applies to the body as well. Your body is changing atoms and molecules (which are subtle energy patterns) at such a rapid rate that you truly are a different person when you wake up in the morning from the one you were when you went to sleep the previous night. You acquire a new stomach lining every five days with the inner most layer of stomach cells exchanged in a matter of minutes as you digest food. Your skeletal system, seemingly so solid and rigid, is entirely new every three months. Your skin is new every five weeks. The flow of oxygen, carbon, hydrogen, and nitrogen is so rapid you could be a whole new person in a matter of weeks. Maybe the old saying, "A new you is coming through" is not off base. What will really make the difference for the "new you" emerging is not found outside yourself, but rather deep inside.

You appear to be the same outwardly, yet you are like a building whose bricks are constantly being replaced by new ones. Every year, 98 percent of the total number of atoms (your building blocks) in your body are fully replaced. This is not just a thought or theory; it's the natural law of particulate matter. This amazing fact about the body has been validated by radioisotope studies at the Oak Ridge Laboratories in California. Thoughts, beliefs, and emotions influence the atoms that comprise your body. You can begin to see small imbalances in your subtle energy patterns; the effects these shifts have on our body sow the seeds of future symptoms, illness, and disease. Conversely, bringing microscopic imbalances back into balance (harmony) will set the stage for a future of health and a life of fulfillment.

When I was at a point in developing a way to interpret this subtle energy language and how it would be useful in healing, I was fortunate enough to have a combination of my earlier trainings fall into place in unusual ways. I began to see the entire body in relationship to all of the space around it. The body became a reference point in time. I had to start with an anatomical reference of anterior (front), posterior (back), left side and right side, headward and foot-ward. I realized if I was going to understand the body stories that the subtle energies were giving me as a healer, I had to understand the geography of the body from an emotions roadmap. My training in Neurolinguistic programming (NLP) had taught me that emotionally our brains think in timelines. Often in working with clients, I would have them stand on an imaginary timeline. Facing forward became in their mental/emotional reference their future. Behind them became their "past." This was true of left and right as well. (Left became the past and right became their future as points of reference in time when dealing with mental/emotional issues.)

Congruent with this training and reinforcing the appropriate approach, I remembered from my own personal growth experiences what my mentors had taught me about my body in relationship to time and space. When I was first emerging into my studies of metaphysics, my friends and mentors, Leon and his wife Mary, introduced me to many things; however, one of the most intriguing was Grandfather Jack, who was a 100-plus year old Hopi Indian Medicine man to whom Leon introduced me in the Arizona desert outside of Sedona. Grandfather Jack solidified for me what I had studied in other indigenous cultures, which also correlated with the Native American culture.

He helped me understand that our body is a place of unity between all aspects of the Universe and we integrate these universal energies as well as experiences through our physical experience on this planet. He taught that if we think of the body as a place of unity, then energy flows from above (Father Sky in spirit world) and is where energy enters the body. The energy moves through our body towards our center. Also in this unity, energy that flows from below, or Mother Earth, also extends energy from the ground. This energy moves from our feet to the center of our body, allowing for a comingling of these energies deep inside our bodies. These co-mingled energies are the inner expression of us out in the world. Remarkably, this fits my chiropractic principles that state that the nervous system operates in the world from the concept of above, down, inside, and out. In other words, the flow of energy in the body goes from the brain (above) down (through the spinal cord) and from inside (the central nervous system) out (through the spinal and peripheral nerves) to every cell, tissue, and organ in the body. To make a long process of epiphanies a shorter story, I developed a geographic emotional map of how I felt the body could give us stories that might help us heal more completely.

It is essential to note that the correlations I make in this model of looking at the body-mind are not at all linear, but are expressions of disharmonies in our subtle energy patterns. Taking into account these disharmonies in the energy flow of the body, I discovered that we could start building a story by looking at left-sided pain/problems and right-sided pain/problems. A general rule based on the model here in this book is left-sided problems anywhere in the body tend to indicate issues from the past, the feminine, and receiving energies from others. Right-sided problems anywhere in the body tend to be associated with current issues or the anticipation of future events, the masculine, and giving of our energy to others.

For example, let's say you are experiencing neck and shoulder pain on the left side of your body. From the concepts in this book, we can look at the neck as representing the conduit between the head (our cultural or social programming) and the heart (the center of our passions, desires, and intuition). This disharmony may represent feelings of conflict between the heart and the head. There may be feelings of inflexibility if you are experiencing neck stiffness or lack of mobility. If you are feeling a sore throat or tightness in the muscles of the neck, you may be feeling trapped by a situation or circumstance. Stiff muscles in the neck may also be a representation of not being able to express or take action on your true feelings.

If there is a conflict in our life between what we feel in our heart is the intuitive thing to do and that conflicting voice in our head saying, "You can't do that" or "No one will let you be that way," then this conflict will exhibit itself in the neck in the form of tension in our physical body. Dr. Mario Martinez, clinical neuropsychologist, agrees with *Longevity, and Success*, wherein he describes the neck as the place where we process expression versus suppression. He states that the neck and shoulders represent the balance between the ability (or freedom) to express ourselves versus the suppression of our expression from within ourselves or by others around us. We may experience tension here when we need to express something and are not doing so. Shoulders are often associated with carrying a burden of the conflict between our heart's desires and the head's rational, cultural programmed suppression.

What I learned in clinical practice was that I could create a non-linear story that brings all of these energy disharmonies together in the form of a Health Code. With this defined, we could explore the idea that something in a client's current environment is stimulating the memory of an experience from their past. In this past experience they felt trapped and couldn't express their true feelings. Another way to state this is that in your past something created a burden for you. This burden may have made your life feel inflexible. This burden made you think or feel that you had limited choices about how to take action. You ultimately chose to suppress rather than express your feelings about it. This may have led to a behavior you are continuing to do that is blocking your ability to truly live from your heart. Perhaps someone in your past has told you that you can't have what you truly want. Maybe you feel disempowered and so you feel like you are "not enough" to do what you are called to do from your heart and intuition. Get the general idea?

Take Tess as another illustration of the Health Code principles. She is a very talented clothing designer, both young and ambitious. She also was in a serious relationship with who she felt was the man of her dreams. She presented in my office with a nagging right-sided neck and shoulder pain. On examination, I found decreased range of motion especially turning to the right. While doing breathing and soft tissue release, we went through a brain-to-pain process of association.

In that treatment session, she discovered that she was suppressing her own dreams of a successful career in clothing design. She had an opportunity to design in SoHo in New York City. This incredible opportunity would potentially launch her new clothing line. She realized that her fear was that she was choosing her career over her dream relationship. This burden of the conflict between her head and her heart represented by pain and muscle tension in the neck and shoulders was now more apparent to her. The pain of possibly suppressing her creative expression (right shoulder) versus the pain of passing up the man of her dreams (her heart) was generating tension in her neck, which was the channel of communication (conflict, in this case) between her head and her heart. Ultimately, she made the choice to follow her creative process and honor her own genius. Her pain subsided a few days after our session as she became aware and clear regarding what decision was most appropriate for her. She is extremely successful to this day.

In my work exploring the insights and stories being expressed in your Health Code, it is important to understand the interrelationship of all systems: the physical systems as well as the subtle energy systems that operate within the body. These subtle communications with the physiological systems by way of the neurological, fascial, chakra, hormonal (endocrine), and acupuncture systems solidified my seven gateways concept into a usable form. I researched ways to make sense of how these different systems communicate, and this tactic also gave my model of healing a way to understand the whole body-mind system.

For most people when it comes to "energy healing," they are most commonly familiar with the chakra system. A brief review may be helpful, even if you are aware of chakras. Though around and acknowledged by various cultures for centuries, most authorities describe chakras as swirling wheels of energy that correspond to massive nerve centers in the body. Each of the seven main chakras contain bundles of nerves that relate to major organs which process and influence our psychological, emotional, and spiritual states of being. Since everything is moving energetically throughout the body and all of our systems, it is essential that our seven chakras and our seven bioemotional gateways stay open, aligned in harmony with each other, and remain fluid. If there is a blockage in a center or multiple centers, energy flow and communication between systems becomes restricted.

Think of something as simple as your bathtub drain. If you allow too much hair to go into the drain, the bathtub will back up with water, stagnate, and eventually bacteria or mold will grow. So it is, too, with our bodies using the chakras and bio-emotional gateways. A bathtub is a simple fix. Keeping the chakras and gateways open is a bit more challenging. Currently, most books on chakras relate each one to a particular endocrine gland and there is a fair amount of agreement across authors concerning these relationships. So we consider it fairly common knowledge concerning chakra-endocrine relationships. On the other hand, there is little written about the details of chakra-neuro-plexuses relationships, even though many authors make a point to mention that such a relationship exists. Relationship isn't always strictly about anatomy; it is more often about how the mind, body, and spirit functionally relate and integrate. When we consider that organs within the endocrine system talk to the central nervous system (spine) and peripheral nervous system (nerves) as readily as the opposite, it seems simple. The organs of the endocrine system that have a well-established relationship with the chakra system are linked to the acupuncture system and the nerve plexuses to the central nervous system.

To create a clearer picture, the seven main chakras are aligned along the spine; they start at the base and finish at the top of the head and are portals passing entirely through the body at their appropriate location. As these energies flow as I noted earlier, they pass through nerve plexuses. Since we are dealing with energy and healing, it's important to remember a basic energy principle from physics. Subtle energy can rotate at different speeds; the size of the energy field may vary. The intensity of the energy (color) may vary. This holds true with chakras and is influenced by a person's personal growth, physical condition, energy levels, disease, and/ or stress. The nerve plexuses sense these changes and variants in energy and either register them as harmony or disharmony to the whole body.

The chakras themselves are focused on different aspects of living. The lower three chakras (or bio-emotional gateways) are associated with meeting your basic needs like food, sex, shelter, and money. The three upper-most are associated with more spiritual pursuits such as evolving, finding purpose, meaning, and contributing to the world. The middle chakra (heart chakra), the Love Gateway, balances the lower and upper chakras to achieve harmony in the mind, body, and spirit. If a chakra/gateway becomes imbalanced or blocked, it can manifest as illness, emotional upset or distress, and this disharmony allows diseases to develop. The chakras/gateways become blocked/imbalanced by negative energy, repressed emotions, toxins such as drugs, alcohol, and corn chips, as well as from traumatic experiences.

Most practitioners of acupuncture and Asian medicine in the Americas, Europe, and Australia tend to regard this style of energy healing as originating in China. However, when exploring the numerous healing disciplines from scores of nations, the topic of chakras as it relates to acupuncture and healing becomes a challenge due to the extreme amount of knowledge from all these different cultures and geographic areas. They include regions we would not normally consider, like Syria, Turkey, Iran, Afghanistan, and Pakistan, along with ancient Greece and Rome. The healing philosophies of Persia and India also had an extremely strong influence on our understanding of how the acupuncture, nervous system, and chakras are related.

There is a strong correlation between the caduceus symbol adopted by Western medicine and the Indian medicine symbols of ida, pingala, and sushumna. This helps explain the effect of energies and how we can understand and apply healing. The caduceus is a single staff with two snakes double-coiled around it. The sushumna, the staff, represents the power centers of the body as the spinal tracts (nerve tracts or pathways of the central nervous system). The snakes are twisting around the staff and are, referred to as the ida and pingala. The ida represents yin energy, which is considered negative, internal and feminine. Sorry women. The pingala represents the yang energy, which is considered positive, external and masculine. Every time the ida and pingala cross one another, that crossing forms a chakra when the staff is visualized as the body.

Historically, these chakras are represented on the front of a body diagram. When we combine the chakras with the bio-emotional gateways, there is a correlation with what we know in acupuncture as Conception Vessel and Governing Vessel acupoints. Since the gateways are portals through the body, each gateway has a specific relationship to a particular vertebral level on the back of the body. Linking the nerve plexus of that area with the acupuncture meridian influence can engage one of the most powerful healing effects. For example, the 5th chakra, The Expression Gateway, is connected with the acupuncture point between C7/T1 (the last cervical vertebrae and the first thoracic vertebrae). We have learned clinically to make a correlation between the involved acupoints, the nerve plexus and the associated chakra—what we call bio-emotional gateways. Therapeutically we can use acupoint locations on the front and back of the body related to the involved gateway. These gateways create communication between all systems and allow us access to deep bio-emotional healing. This emotional healing will bring balance back to multiple systems within the body at one time.

Although the chakra system is an ancient discovery and the emotional gateway system is more modern science, both are contributing to a deeper understanding when it comes to healing. We are constantly learning how these systems can affect the outcomes we experience in our bodies, our lives, and in our overall wellness. The chakra "gateways" are the interplay of endocrine, acupuncture, energy, emotions, and central nervous system communication locations. The endocrine system alone affects almost every organ and cell in the body. The endocrine system produces hormones that regulate our metabolism, growth and development, tissue function, sexual function, reproduction, sleep, and mood. When energy is blocked or stuck in one of the bioemotional gateways, the functioning of the corresponding gland may be altered. The nervous system function will be altered and the acupuncture meridians will be altered. Alteration in any or all of these systems will create imbalance in various ways to the body. Each chakra, each one of these bio-emotional gateways, is connected to several organs via the nervous system and acupuncture system. So, when energy is congested in the chakra/gateway, communication can be altered affecting the functioning of the organs. This leaves the doorway open to decreased immune system function and the possibility of disease. It is, therefore, important to keep our chakras balanced, our gateways open, and energy flowing.

Awareness Keys

- We tend to think of our bodies as fixed solid material objects only. In truth they are subtle energy centers constantly changing with our thoughts, emotions, behaviors and the environment surrounding us.

- As body geography goes, remember that anything left-sided is related to your past. Anything right-sided is related to anticipation of future events. Anything above the diaphragm is more spiritual, altruistic related. Anything below the diaphragm is more foundational, grounding or primal related.

- Part of exploring your Health Code is bringing all of the energy disharmonies (symptoms) together in a useful healing non-linear story.

- When memories from our past get triggered from something or someone in our present experience, the physiological cascade of symptoms can begin.

- This cascade of symptoms can become a healing story from our body. It may show us how to forgive ourselves from our past experiences. It may also show us where to let go of our anxiety about the anticipation of our future experiences.

- The point of this is to heal and to return our body-mind to a place of "okay-ness" with the present moment. Knowing that all is "okay" in this moment, frees us to take conscious action and make conscious decisions.

- There are seven main chakras aligned along the spine that allow energy to flow through to the front of the body.

- These chakra centers, which communicate with our nerve-plexuses and acupuncture meridian systems, make up our bio-emotional gateways.

- These seven bio-emotional gateways can become blocked or imbalanced by negative energy, repressed emotions, toxins, or traumatic experiences.

- When we clear our bio-emotional gateways we have an abundant, clear flow of energy in our body-mind. When our bio-emotional gateways are free flowing, we have freedom in our nervous system, chakra system, acupuncture system, and hormonal system.

- As was stated before, these systems are whispering to each other constantly. You can listen, explore, and use these systems for healing.

Chapter 4
Body Roadmap

*The greatest mistake in the treatment of disease is
that there are physicians for the body and physicians
for the soul, although the two cannot be separated.*

Plato

The notion of an integrated body-mind process has a long history in Indigenous, Asian, Middle Eastern cultures, philosophies, and practices throughout the world. Western practice began in the 1930's with the work of Wilhelm Reich, a student of Sigmund Freud. Reich began to understand that neuroses live in the body. He found by working directly on or with the body through touch, breath, and movement, it was possible to cure the patient and to relieve them of symptoms. Elsa Gindler, who developed Sensory Awareness, and Moshé Feldenkrais, the founder of Functional Integration, worked in an attempt to heal themselves from illness or accidents when medical science was unable to help. By healing themselves, these pioneers solidified the idea that turning the attention to the life of our body (somas, from Greek somatikos, which signifies the living, aware, bodily person) gives us the capacity to foster our own healing.

Their breakthrough for the West has spawned many forms of healing. Healing practices such as bodywork, dance therapy, biofeedback, movement therapy, and body-oriented psychotherapy. Many, if not all, of these healing methods have influenced my own approach to healing. This kind of work is growing, and many people are helped by it. I hope this work continues to make a paradigm shift in healing. To work with the body and mind of someone in this way is to work with the wholeness of their being. To do this work, we observe how life is processed in the individual and how the individual responds to life. We then introduce practices of attention, conversation, movement, breathing, and awareness. This type of body-centered coaching/guidance takes into account the whole of the person. This type of coaching opens the energy-injured person to learning about themselves. It empowers owning the role of cultivating the self that allows self-care, self-healing, and self-educating.

In reflecting on the earlier story of Mary and her migraine, we can begin the process of looking deeper into the body's Health Code. There are many ways to organize soma systems. In order to give this some sense of fluidity for myself, I chose to follow the energy and that's how I'll share it here. Energy, as we understand and previously described, moves in its creation from above down and from inside out. When energy flow gets stuck or blocked, it gets stunted in multiple areas. Grandfather Jack shared that energy moves from Father Sky (the heavens) into our physical bodies. The other part of his premise is that energy appears to increase its density in our bodies in a way that allows us to integrate and experience Spirit through matter. This energy flows from our head's 7th crown chakra to our 1st root chakra at the base of our pelvic floor. As a chiropractor and neurological researcher, I think of energy moving from head (brain) through the body by way of the spinal and peripheral nerves to every cell and tissue in the body. Energy animates life in our bodies.

The seven chakras/bio-emotional gateways of the body highlight the connection between energy, the endocrine and nervous systems with their links to all body parts and organs, and wellness. The seven gateways (starting at the head and moving through the organs, glands, and body parts) are covered in this section as a body roadmap. You will notice as you begin to study the influence of these gateways throughout the body that each gateway has a central aspect of energy concentration. It is also important to notice that the gateways are also represented starting with the sixth gateway through the first gateway in the arms and legs. The seventh gateway being our connection to the Universal Life force is not represented in the extremities because of its important connection to our central nervous system. To state this very simply, the upper extremity expresses the energy of the gateways from the shoulder to the hand in the sequence of the sixth gateway to the first gateway. The lower extremity starting at the hip to the feet, expresses the sixth through the first gateways. This will all make sense as you dive into each gateway and its representation in the body roadmap. To begin understanding the inter-relationships, the seven emotional gateways in their simplest form are listed here.

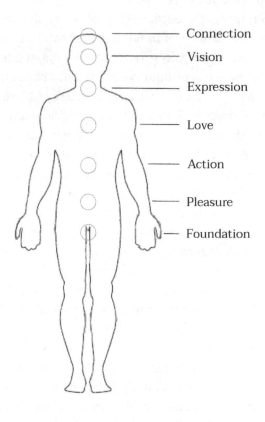

Connection

Vision

Expression

Love

Action

Pleasure

Foundation

Gateways

7th Gateway, The Connection Gateway (crown chakra)
Covers the cerebral cortex, brain stem, and vagus nerve

Head, pituitary gland, and hypothalamus primary; secondarily, the pineal gland, spinal cord; connection to Spirit, the Universe, where we pull information from the stream of consciousness and integrate that energy into our bodies

6th Gateway, The Vision Gateway (third eye chakra)
Covers the carotid plexus

Eyes, brain, specifically the pineal gland and the cerebral cortex; influences the entire central nervous system, shoulders, hips

5th Gateway, The Expression Gateway (throat chakra)
Covers pharyngeal plexus

Thyroid, parathyroid glands, nose, mouth, TMJ, vocal cords, tongue, esophagus, cervical spine, upper arm, thigh

4th Gateway, The Love Gateway (heart chakra)
Covers cardiac plexus

Heart, lungs, thymus gland, upper thoracic spine, elbow, knee

3rd Gateway, The Action Gateway (solar plexus chakra)
Covers celiac or solar plexus

Adrenal, small intestines, pancreas, liver, gallbladder, stomach, lower thoracic spine, muscles, forearm, calf (lower leg)

2nd Gateway, The Pleasure Gateway (sacral plexus chakra
Covers splenic plexus, sacral plexus

Kidney, uterus, bladder, prostate, large intestine, spleen, lumbar spine, ankle, wrist

1st Gateway, The Foundation Gateway (root chakra)
Covers coccygeal plexus

Testes, ovaries, rectum, pelvis, sacrum, bones, hands, feet, spinal cord

Caution for the reader on how this next section is structured: The following information can be overwhelming if taken or consumed in its entirety. It may cause bloating of the mind and even stimulate nausea. It is better digested a small portion at a time. Much like a seven-course meal, take your time and enjoy each part of this section to get the full flavor of the topic. One way to proceed is by considering a symptom or area of discomfort in your own body, then go directly to that section and read about it. See if any of it applies to you specifically. You may want to do this also with a friend or a loved one as a great way to generate some conversation. It is a great way to explore your emotional wellness. You could make it a game to become curious about what might be the hidden emotional quality of the symptoms (imbalanced energy) you are experiencing in your body-mind. As a healing practitioner, once you get a better feel for this material you can work through these concepts with clients. Even something as simple as stating, "You know that your shoulder pain, on an emotional or energetic perspective might be about some feeling that you can't fully express yourself. Can you relate to this anywhere in your life right now?" Then just get quiet, let that resonate with them and usually, they will respond with, "Oh yeah, I know exactly what that is about." At that point, you can use any or a combination of the methods outlined later in the book to help them get in touch with and release the emotional charge that they are carrying in their shoulder. Try it. I think you will be surprised how easy it is to access and heal this emotional energy.

Chapter 5

The Connection Gateway

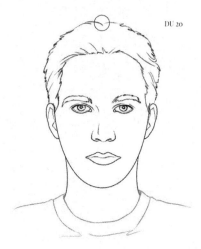

DU 20

The Connection Gateway, also known as the crown chakra, is considered the master control system of the body, so it is a good place to begin our journey. This gateway is located near the top of head and extends to one inch above the eyebrows. Violet is its color. It is the gateway that gives access to higher states of consciousness. It takes us beyond our personal preoccupations and visions. It is where we are able to access the stream of consciousness, the bio-cloud, and our connection to all that exists.

The Connection Gateway is primarily associated with the pituitary gland and hypothalamus; it is secondarily associated to the pineal gland. The hypothalamus and pituitary gland work in tandem to regulate the endocrine system. Because of the location, it is associated with the brain and the whole nervous system. The brain acts as the antenna that is the receptor of information from the constant and continuous flow of the stream of consciousness. I call the stream of consciousness the "bio-cloud" when it relates to our body-mind. Based on how our computers and cell phones interact with "the cloud" most of us understand this metaphor. Current scientific research believes this bio-cloud is where memory is actually stored, much like how the cloud stores data and interacts with our cell phones. In theory, the human energy field (HEF, as discussed earlier) surrounds our body, directly interacting with the stream of consciousness that flows through the Universe. This subtle energy field holds our energy patterns (memories) and our nervous system then picks up the information held there as it responds and adapts to our environment.

These subtle energy systems play an integral part in the total functioning of the human being. It appears from research that the physical system is far from being a closed system. It is only one of several systems that are in dynamic equilibrium from a frequency standpoint. These higher energy systems are actually composed of matter with different frequency characteristics than that of the physical body. There is considerable evidence to suggest that what exists is a holographic energy template associated with the physical body. This etheric body is an energy body that looks quite similar to the physical body over which it is superimposed. The physical body is so energetically connected and dependent upon the etheric body for cellular guidance that the physical body cannot exist without the etheric body. If the etheric field becomes distorted, physical disease soon follows. Many illnesses begin first in the etheric body and are later manifested in the physical body as organ pathology.

Dr. Michael Gerber explains the human subtle energy frequency spectrum like a piano keyboard. It was noted that octaves of musical notes could be seen as similar to octaves of electromagnetic energy. The lowest keys on the left side of the keyboard were compared to the physical spectrum of frequencies. The next step of keys to the right formed the energetic musical scale of the etheric realm. Still further to the right, beyond the frequencies of the etheric, lies the next higher octave of energy frequencies, comparable to the astral realm of matter and energy. This realm is the energy frequencies of the emotions. Although this analogy is thought to extend still further, encompassing a full seven octaves of higher frequency levels. But we will stop here. If you have not been exposed to this thinking, I feel it is important to be exposed to this as a healer, coach and practitioner.

I include the spinal cord in this because the Connection Gateway, the seventh (crown) chakra, has a connection with the Foundation Gateway, the first (root) chakra as they are both at the ends of the central nervous system connected by the spinal cord. If you are a healer that uses cranial sacral technique or a yoga instructor and healer that works with Kundalini energy, you will be familiar with this connection between the first and seventh gateways. My chiropractic and osteopathic colleagues are also familiar with the cranial sacral pump that exists in the physical body to move and circulate the cerebral spinal fluid.

This gateway, when imbalanced, can manifest as: being disconnected to spirit, constant cynicism regarding what is sacred, living in your head, being disconnected from your body and/or matters of reality, and could manifest as closed-mindedness.

There are several physical components of this gateway that can hold blocked impressions and show manifestations of blocked energy.

The Head: Cranium

The head involves a variety of things, but for simplicity's sake we will talk about headaches. Headaches get a lot of press, don't they? Name at least three well-televised medication commercials for relief of head pain. If that took more than 30 seconds to answer, it would be surprising. It shows you the "common" headache is common. Therefore, knowing that headaches are a prolific problem in our society, one might wonder what this could possibly mean on an emotional level.

Headaches can have many forms that may come from many different primary causes. You may not know that headaches that don't involve a primary cause are extremely uncommon. Confusion and feeling overwhelmed are the two most common feelings associated with headaches of an emotional nature. Primarily these headaches are caused by muscle tension. Other common primary causes are hormone fluctuations, liver toxicity, high and low blood sugar levels, bowel toxicity or sluggishness, sinus infections, food sensitivities, and environmental allergies.

Headaches are complex and may need professional interpretation in determining the primary cause or factors. Many of you healers may practice functional medicine or some form of nutritional consultation and you will want to continue to explore these primary causes with your clients. However, in conjunction with discovering the primary cause, we can use this process to explore what emotions might be contributing to our symptoms. This is right in line with how muscle tension generated by stressful emotional stimulations can lead to many of our common headaches. Reduce the stress, release the emotional energy that is causing the tension, and the headaches resolve.

Here is another thought. Let's say the primary cause of your headache is a food sensitivity or food allergy. Emotionally, you would look at how well you are digesting even taking in new information or new "food for thought." If you are being confronted with new ideas, you may be feeling frustrated or overwhelmed. Looking at emotions is important. However, if the primary cause is food allergies or sensitivity, then a comprehensive approach is the best. A thorough approach would include evaluating liver toxicity from eating processed, preservative-laden foods, drinking excesses of alcohol, or from social or prescription drug use. The potential protocol you would want to follow would be consulting with a nutritionist about a liver detoxification program. You could also choose to make some healthy lifestyle changes around your food choices and medication management. But, this book is not about those approaches. So, looking at the emotional component associated with the liver, you would want to question where in your life you have unresolved anger and resentment.

This is how another type of emotional investigation may proceed. Jen was a new patient and she had chronic headaches. On examination I found neck tension, decreased range of motion in the cervical spine as well as low functioning frontal and cerebellar brain activity. These are common when the brain is under stress and is suffering from early signs of poor brain function due to inflammation and poor blood sugar regulation in the body. I wanted to make sure that Jen was receiving a comprehensive approach to her headache challenge. We did comprehensive blood work, and I won't bore you with the results here. But we found blood sugar regulation to be off as well as many inflammatory markers indicating she would need to change her diet and lifestyle. I made sure to reduce her muscle tension with soft tissue work, restored motion to the cervical spine, and we worked on the emotional components involved.

She was in the midst of a potential change in job, geographic move, and a shift in her relationship. Now I'm not sure if you feel this way, but this is the perfect storm for an abundance of confusion. We worked through each decision and gave her homework that helped her take the confusion out of her life and her mind. She became clearer about what decisions to make and how to honor her path in life. We helped her get in touch with the best choices she could make so that she could utilize all of her gifts, talents, and abilities. She made the changes in her diet and she began to find the priority of exercise, rest, and relaxation in her life. She balanced many different aspects of her life, relationship and career. She made herself the central concern in getting well. By honoring herself, much of the confusion and overwhelm was released.

You have seen with Jen's and also with Mary's story how headaches can block the energy of the connection gateway. Another example of this was with Sammy who came to me with a history of headaches. I questioned her about the areas of lifestyle just as I did in Jen's case. However, she was, by most standards, the epitome of health in that she had a great diet, she was allergy aware, exercised daily, slept well, and was hormonally balanced. On further questioning, what came up for her around stressors in her life were overwhelm in work and relationship as well as confusion about career. You see many of us experience work-related stress but are okay in knowing we are moving forward in our long-term careers. Think about this—stress about money versus stress about finances. These differences in our language seem small, but in our emotional wellbeing they can be large. I won't go deeper into this now, but simply, work is our day-to-day job task, as money is our day-to-day utilization of our resources.

Career is our intention of what we are doing long term with our life, as is our financial wellbeing. Both have stress attached to them, but making the correct distinction between these stresses can lead us to different stuck or blocked emotions. Sammy was stuck in her day to day and was feeling overwhelmed and confused. The tension of this stress and her drive to make her life meaningful got blocked or stuck in her Connection Gateway. I worked with her with soft tissue release and had her perform deep breath work through a visualization as I held points to open her Connection Gateway. Through the visualization process I helped her see that she had lost her connection to the stream of consciousness that is her guiding principle of life. She began to redefine her perspective on her "big picture." She realized there was a gap between where she is currently and where she is hoping to be long term. Together we examined the gap between these two things and noticed that it was much bigger in her imagination than in reality. When she thought the space and time between these was big, it would make her anxious, thinking she would never get there. With this came tension in her head, neck, jaw, and shoulders. Once she realized that this distance between these two things was not in reality that far, she began to let go of the overwhelm. She was able to release the overwhelm of never achieving her goals. She released the tension in her head associated with the confusion about trying to mentally make things different. She ended the sessions knowing that she could be relaxed, keep moving along the course of her current life and that she was actually right on track with her goals. She got off the table without her headache. She was also free of the critical voice in her head. She was able to replace her overwhelm and confusion with a feeling of peace, joy, and grace about the process of life just as it is.

As students of the Health Code model, you begin to see the endless possibilities here. I remember in school one of my professors authored a book titled *Anything Can Cause Anything*. It is now apparent to me how true this rings. A cycle is often established in the body-mind where if you are angry, your anger will create a toxic liver. It is true that if your liver is in a toxic state that this will lead to more feelings of anger, even encourage an angry personality. Often anger will provoke a person to drink alcohol or use drugs to diminish the anger, which creates a more toxic liver leading to more anger. There are many of these downward spiraling cycles in the body-mind. You cannot just look at the symptoms without looking at the whole picture of what is going on in a person's life. Oh, and by the way, regardless of what television commercials have told you, THERE IS NO SUCH THING AS A NORMAL HEADACHE! Headaches, no matter your perspective, are not normal.

Pituitary Gland (The Master Hormonal Gland)

The pituitary gland is well known for its function of hormonal feedback to the other organs of the body. In a sense, it's like the quarterback of the organ systems. It has the supreme purpose of monitoring the levels of a variety of hormones in the blood stream, then stimulating either an increase or decrease of needed hormones in the blood. This is a very simplistic approach to an incredibly sophisticated and complicated system, but I am not trying to teach you to be an endocrinologist or physiologist. I would hope that what I have said would just imprint in your mind the basic function of this organ/gland.

From the more esoteric perspective of the chakras, the function of the Connection Gateway is to draw source energy to keep the spiritual, mental, emotional, and physical health of the body in balance. When I was working with and researching these emotional gateways in connection with glands, I discovered it once again comes down to energy and harmony. Disturbances in subtle energy of the gateways translate into physical manifestation and symptoms that are associated with the corresponding gland and organs. Emotional gateways, remember, are energy centers that influence our being at many levels.

From the Health Code concept, the pituitary gland has to do with the following emotions: non-thinking, non-emotive (that feeling of being checked out, present physically but absent mentally/emotionally), depleted, suppressed, sluggish memory, can't-get-it-together feeling. So the hide and seek game that a person is doing in their life is played out within the pituitary gland. This happens when the person's behavior towards others is not straightforward and they pretend to be someone they are not. This occurs when the person refuses to respect their intuition. As I stated previously, the 6th and 7th emotional gateways traditionally include both the pineal and pituitary glands, partly because of their anatomical proximity. However, in this book we will consider the pineal gland to be associated with the 6th gateway, the Vision Gateway, the third eye chakra located at the brow center.

Awareness Keys

- When you think of anything pertaining to the head, always think emotionally that it could be related to overwhelm, confusion, or a disconnect from our spiritual connection.

- When someone is struggling with hormonal issues, another thought could be that the pituitary gland is blocked, or there are unresolved emotions stuck there. Some of those emotions to explore are where is the person feeling suppressed, depleted, or having a hard time "getting it together"?

Chapter 6
The Vision Gateway

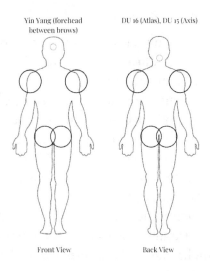

Yin Yang (forehead between brows)

DU 16 (Atlas), DU 15 (Axis)

Front View

Back View

The Vision Gateway is above and between the eyes, with indigo or purple as its color. It is the gateway driven by the principle of openness and imagination. It is said to be where the duality of a personal "I" is separate from the rest of the world, where our personality exists independently from everything else. This gateway is associated with the pineal gland, which is in charge of regulating biorhythms, including activities like sleep and wake time, but also the rhythms of our lives and how things flow from one thing to the next. It is related to perception and altered or mystical states of consciousness. It is also related to these behavioral and psychological characteristics: vision, intuition, perception of subtle dimensions, and movement of energy. This gateway gives access to mystical states; it connects us to wisdom and insight, motivates inspiration as well as creativity. It helps us perceive the subtle qualities of reality.

The Vision Gateway imbalance can manifest as feeling stuck in the daily grind without being able to look beyond our problems or the inability to set a plan or guiding vision for ourselves. It can be where we get lost in fantasies that appear more real than reality. It often manifests in not being able to establish a vision for oneself and then realize it. It exhibits as a lack of clarity and not seeing the big picture.

Pineal Gland (The Third Eye)

The pineal gland has now been demonstrated to be a gland of major regulatory importance. It regulates the adrenal glands, pancreas, parathyroid gland, and the sex organs. In general, the pineal gland's secretions are inhibitory. It transfers its secretions through the cerebral spinal fluid via the cranial sacral rhythms and breath. The cranial sacral movement as stated earlier is the mechanism that moves cerebral spinal fluid in the body. We know that the pineal gland secretions also move through the circulatory system as well. The pineal gland responds to light and dark cycles, daylight and nighttime, circadian rhythms, and other cyclic behavior in our environment as well as in the body. Its secretions regulate some familiar neuro-hormones like melatonin and serotonin levels in the brain and body.

In the Health Code, then, the pineal gland is associated with being in our natural rhythm, being in a balanced state, and flowing with our natural cycles. So, the emotions of being overwhelmed, feeling that life is out of balance, and a sense of loss of vision in life are common emotions associated with pineal stress. This gateway allows access to the utmost clarity and wisdom. When this gateway is imbalanced, it can manifest emotionally and psychologically as being disconnected to spirit, with constant cynicism regarding what is sacred. The exact opposite side of this is an overactive connection in the Vision Gateway and can be linked in part to the technology saturation in our world today.

Since the two (both the Connection Gateway and the Vision Gateway) are somewhat linked through the relationship of the pituitary and pineal glands, the results that manifest in this condition are defined by being disconnected from your body along with close-mindedness. The way to return balance to this vital organ can be taking more time for meditation, prayer, yoga, Tai Chi, exercise, or simply slowing down to smell the roses. Often, tactics of just returning to a more normal cycle of life, such as going to sleep at a reasonable hour, getting proper wake-sleep cycles established, waking up early enough to meditate, contemplate or exercise and nourishing the body before running off into our hectic lifestyle, will work wonders on improving the function of the pineal gland.

These activities are beneficial in decreasing feelings of being overwhelmed and tend to be proactive in returning balance to life. I highly recommend you find a way to apply the Eleven Principles of Nature in your life. Robert Williams, the developer of Psych–K, and Bruce Heinemann, a nature photographer, collaborated to outline the Eleven Principles of Nature in a beautiful way. Though you'll be able to glean more by using information in the reference section of this book, consider the simplicity of this list and how you can improve your processes with clarity like this.

He states these eleven principles as the following:

1. Collaboration – not competition

2. Adaptation

3. Diversity

4. Harmony

5. Cause and Effect

6. Resiliency

7. Balance

8. Interconnectedness

9. Timing

10. Enough is enough/More is not always better

11. Effective use of Resources

The Vision Gateway is associated with emotional and psychological characteristics, connection to wisdom and insight, motivation, inspiration, and creativity. This gateway helps us be able to perceive subtle energy and dimensions. It may help with psychic abilities related to clairvoyance and clairaudience, illumination and vision.

When the Vision Gateway is imbalanced, it can give you the feeling of being stuck in the daily grind without being able to look beyond your problems and set a guiding vision for yourself. It may manifest as fantasies that appear more real than reality. You may not be able to see the greater picture or you may lack clarity about your direction in life.

The Shoulder

The shoulder occupies a geographic location in the body that overlaps the Vision Gateway and interacts with the Expression Gateway. (Similarly, the hip is a unique area of emotional influence between two gateways/chakras.) Since the shoulder is associated with the emotions of the Vision Gateway and shares the energy of the emotions of the Expression Gateway, this can give rise to a more complex emotional story in some cases.

There is a familiar lamentation about carrying the "weight of the world on your shoulders." Included in this shoulder scenario is the concept of how you are expressing yourself. The shoulder is classically associated with the body insight of holding onto something that needs to be said but is not getting said or expressed. It may also manifest as having a vision for your life that you cannot find a way to express. There may be something that you are holding back or suppressing. This "thing" then, becomes a burden that you choose to carry around with you. Let's call it a chip. Walking around with a "chip on your shoulder" is not a new concept. However, it is not just a cliché either. In short, the shoulder is about carrying the weight of the world on your shoulders. The shoulder can represent not expressing a vision of your life that needs to be expressed. Your shoulders may be carrying resentment about this or a chip from your past. Shoulder tension may represent the emotion of you waiting for an opportunity or permission to express your deeply held feelings rather than continue to suppress those feelings. See how this gets blocked in the shoulders, festers, and continues to manifest in pain?

If you can find the voice to cut it all loose in a safe way with your thoughts, then you can release the pressure off your system and feel the relief of expressing yourself. In addition, there are the feelings of grief and sadness associated with the shoulders. Frequently the grief or sadness isn't about a situation, but rather from that long suppression of not expressing your deepest feelings. And you thought a shoulder was just a shoulder.

Clinical research highlights how this works. An example illustrated by my friend, colleague, and esteemed healer, Evy Cugelman, RN, is a good case. Evy is a highly trained nurse and therapeutic touch practitioner as well as a therapeutic touch educator and trainer. Her client, Nancy, was involved in an auto accident in which she experienced a minor whiplash injury and sustained injuries to her neck and upper trapezius muscles, ligaments, and tendons. She exhibited muscle spasms, pain, and inflammation as a result. Twenty years prior to coming to see Evy, Nancy had been the victim of an assault and sexual abuse where she had experienced head and neck injuries similar to a whiplash injury. She had healed from these initial injuries due to the assault and had not had a recurrence of her pain since that time.

Again, we are learning over time how crafty the body-mind is to help us resolve these deeper memories. Twenty years later, she was involved in this minor auto accident with a man (the other driver) who reminded her of her abuser in his appearance and his mannerisms. After the encounter, throughout the evening and into the next day she began to experience the original neck and upper trapezius pain from her prior assault and sexual abuse. She realized she had done nothing to generate this level of pain and that the trigger for her was the memory of her original abuser.

She went to Evy for some healing. Evy had a thermographic study done prior to treatment of both TT (therapeutic touch) and then CIM (creative imaging method), the method I use and teach to help clients and other therapists to work through emotional issues. Thermography shows areas of varied colors depending on the heat being generated by the tissues photographed. White, red, orange, and blue indicate gradations of heat and inflammation or cooling of specific tissues. In this case specifically, Nancy's neck, face, and upper trapezius regions are the areas of pain and suspected trauma that were imaged. In the initial thermographic photos before treatment, it was evident that Nancy's neck, face, upper trapezius (shoulders) were represented as highly inflamed. These imaged areas were showing a great amount of white (very inflamed) to red (moderately inflamed) and orange (mildly inflamed). In the photos that followed her therapeutic sessions, where she was taken through first a TT (therapeutic touch) treatment, there was a shift in colors. The shift in colors showed a nice reduction of some of the white areas (most inflamed) and more yellow (less inflamed) and some expansion of blue areas (complete cooling) of tissues after TT.

Following the TT session, Nancy was treated to a session of emotional clearing, called creative imaging method or CIM. Evy did this to release the emotional memory of her previous traumatic experiences, both earlier in her life and the later incident of her auto accident. (CIM is the name I originally gave and used in my earlier teachings for doing a method of emotional release. Over the past two decades this holistic approach became the Health Code.) After this treatment, on the thermography there was a large reduction of some of the remaining white areas (most inflamed). Also, there was less yellow and some expansion of blue areas. There was also a reduction of the red and orange throughout with more greens and blues indicating cooling of the tissues and healing beginning at the tissue level. This occurred nearly immediately, with reduction of pain and inflammation, for the patient. This indicates the removal of the traumatic charge that the patient has been carrying in her neurology since her earlier assault.

This is validated proof of the power of emotional and energy healing along with the associated tissue and chemical changes that take place in the body when appropriate therapies are applied. If you have old trauma and are still having pain, it can be beneficial to take steps to heal the emotional aspect of those events. Those events, circumstances, or memories that occurred during or around the time of a traumatic event are still unresolved and being stored in your tissues. Admitting that emotions do affect the physiology of pain and inflammation in the tissues of the body is a first step. Once you identify that there are emotions, thoughts, feelings, or beliefs that were part of the traumatic event then you can take the next step to healing.

So, what is the best thing to do about it? Start by expressing in some safe way about what is bothering you. Get it out. I already know what you're going to say. "But what I have to say I could never say to the person's face!" So, don't say it to them, do it some other way. Here are a couple of suggestions.

- Go into a quiet room where you can be alone. Put an empty chair in front of you and pretend or visualize that the person to whom you need to express your deeper feelings is sitting in that chair right in front of you. Then, begin by telling them exactly how you feel about what it is you have been carrying around with you for so long. Express how it feels to you emotionally and physically. Let yourself drop into the situation as if it were real and just let it roll. Say everything you have ever wanted to say but didn't have the power or your voice to say it. You will notice that the pace will pick up and before you know it you will be letting it rip. This is an incredible way to process the unresolved emotion in a safe and effective manner.

- An additional or alternate way of doing the same thing is to journal or write a letter about what is troubling you to this person. This process is covered in the 'Say it, burn it, love it!' exercises later in the book. Go for it. Just a little clue for those of you who haven't figured it out yet. All the emotion that you are holding onto in your body about some situation, circumstance, or trauma is only hurting you. The person it is about or directed toward really isn't feeling a thing. They have all of their own crap. They have not given your stuff even one moment of thought. Sorry, but it is the truth.

Buttock and Hip Joint

Beginning with the buttock area, which technically can be considered the hip area, can we imagine that pain in this area might relate literally to the cliché "who is the pain in the butt?" When I have presented this question to a number of clients in the past in a curious manner, they have always responded in an affirmative way and immediately produced someone's name. With this in mind, I began to see that the old cliché actually has validity.

The Vision Gateway also affects the lower extremities, including the buttock and hip joint. However, like the shoulder, this area is an overlap region between the gateways of the central body and the gateways of the lower limb as it attaches to the body. With this overlap, the mixing of bio-emotional energies can easily add to the story the body is trying to tell us.

The buttock area from an insight perspective has been associated with sexual frustration or lack of sexual fulfillment. But, of course, that is not all. I have found the right cheek or buttock to be associated with financial stress, as well as financial trauma or lack of financial fulfillment. Is this combination representative of the cliché "money can't buy you love?" The left cheek or buttock has most commonly been associated with emotional trauma. Specifically early (childhood) emotional or sexual trauma. The whole pelvic region is commonly associated with a variety of sexual issues: sexual abuse or trauma, feeling impotent to make things happen or lack of sexual fulfillment. It often relates to feelings of loss of personal power, and not feeling a strong sense of self. I even find this area relates to clients giving too much to others and not taking care of their own needs, which then manifests as blocked energy here.

More lateral in the pelvis, the actual hip joint area is, like the shoulder, about not expressing yourself. Often, in this particular area since it is so closely associated with the pelvis and all of its various insights, one could conclude that there are many possible Health Code stories. For example, maybe festering energy around sexual trauma, loss of personal power, and the behavior of giving too much to others. Maybe there is blocked energy around feeling of loss of personal power and the inability to feel deserving of financial success or abundance. Perhaps there is a feeling of not being sexually fulfilled for some reason, yet not feeling comfortable about expressing this unfulfilled feeling. In patients presenting to my office, one thing that can significantly affect sexual activity is pain in the low back, pelvis, or hips. This could be one way of avoiding the issue without having to communicate about it. An example might be "Oh, not tonight honey, my back is hurting." Now isn't that ideal for not having to talk about it and not having to process the emotional pain? However, there might be some better and more direct ways of solving this problem.

I have seen in my office the development of hip, low back, or pelvic pain in women who have a child about the age they were when they first experienced sexual trauma. Usually it is a child of the same gender and as the child moves into the age of when the originating event happened in the mother's life, problems emerge. The sequence of events of her child aging will actually open portals to her own memories of experiences at that age, whether conscious or not. This will often reveal itself by the mother developing pain during the mere act of making love to her husband or partner. Now, logically, she knows her husband or partner is not the perpetrator, nor is she back at the age of her trauma. However, the body's memories want to be processed and this may just be the avenue the body chooses to try its very best to resolve the traumatic past. Once the issue (memory) is brought to the surface, processed, and released, the person feels an intense sense of freedom unlike anything they have ever experienced before.

Consider my client, Jane. She was 41 years old and in a new relationship and excited and curious about exploring the relationship with her partner. She was also looking forward to rediscovering her sexual energy. When she came to me, she was depressed about developing hip pain and low back pain. She said the pain was beginning to interfere with her enjoyment of sex with her partner. We began a body centered visualization process that took her back to a time when she was young and curious in her life around sex. She realized that she had allowed her curiosity to put herself in a bad situation. Ultimately, a young man had taken advantage of her. This implanted a belief in her mind that curiosity equals being taken advantage of, and for her, curiosity also equals loss of power.

During the body-centered visualization, she took full responsibility for her part in letting her curiosity put her in a bad position. In that moment in my office, she realized that curiosity is okay. Curiosity is a good thing and won't always put you in harm's way. She then healed her resentment toward the young man that took advantage of her, finding a level of forgiveness for him and for herself in regard to her part in the experience. Jane returned a few weeks later and said, "Hey, doc. My pain is gone and guess what? I'm still exploring my curious side." Another happy story.

The lower area of the brain stem connects our head to the rest of the body, through the cervical spinal cord and the cervical spine. It also makes the connection of the Vision Gateway with the Expression Gateway. This is always an interesting place for emotional healing. Vision and expression of your vision. Hmm, anyone ever get stuck in this issue? It may be the next gateway that actually has the blockage.

Awareness Keys

- The pineal gland is emotionally about being in our natural rhythm, being in a balanced state and going with the flow.

- Common emotions of feeling out of balance or a sense that you have lost your vision/purpose are common with the Vision Gateway and pineal gland blocks.

- The Vision Gateway can be overactive and blocked due to technology saturation.

- The Vision Gateway blocks can result in a person feeling disconnected from their body or closed-minded.

- Possible activities to balance the Vision Gateway are meditation, prayer, yoga, Tai Chi, slowing down, and getting more rest.

- Shoulders are a combination of the Vision and Expression Gateways.

- Shoulders emotionally are about holding onto something that you need to express but didn't or haven't.

Chapter 7

The Expression Gateway

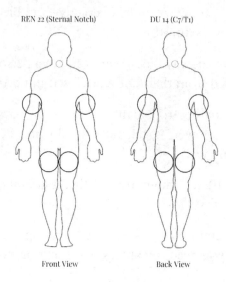

REN 22 (Sternal Notch)   DU 14 (C7/T1)

Front View   Back View

The Expression Gateway has a parallel with the throat chakra, as it is around your vocal cords and the immediate vicinity above and below them. It includes the nose, mouth, and the jaw joint. It carries a blue color. It is the conduit between the lower body and the head. This gateway is driven by the principle of expression and communication. The voice is the element of sound that comes from this gateway. Sound propagates into the air as vibration and can be heard by the ears, but also resonates in our whole body.

The Expression Gateway is associated with the following behavioral and psychological characteristics: expression, especially the ability to express your truth, to speak out, and to have a voice. The Expression Gateway is all about communication, whether it's verbal or non-verbal, external or internal. It is related to turning creative ideas and blueprints into reality. This gateway is where we manifest our vocation, purpose, and a sense of timing. The Expression Gateway, though, has its emphasis on expressing and projecting the creativity into the world according to its perfect form or authenticity.

An imbalance at the throat can manifest as a lack of control over one's speech, speaking too much, or speaking inappropriately. Imbalance manifests as not being able to listen to others, fear of speaking up, having a quiet or imperceptible voice. The Expression Gateway exhibits blockages as not being able to keep secrets, telling lies, or withholding from others. A block here can exhibit as a lack of connection with your vocation or purpose in life.

The Neck, Cervical Spine

This is an interesting emotional area for many reasons. One, the neck has a lot of insights that can be derived from it. Two, neck pain is the second most common complaint that people have (the winning complaint is low back pain: 80 million reported cases per year). That being said, it is obviously an area where many of us get our emotions locked up and are not processing them. One very common phrase heard in our culture is, "So-and-so is such a pain in the neck" or "having to do this @#!*#@ thing is a pain in the neck!"

Patty is a wonderful patient who came to me complaining of neck pain and stiffness with decreased range of motion. After evaluation, I began treating her soft tissues to help release the muscle tension she was experiencing. As I was releasing the tension, I began to have her go into a gentle state of meditation using contemplation and breathing. Knowing that the neck, the Expression Gateway, is a conduit between the heart energy and the head energy, I chose to prompt possible issues. You see, we live in a balance of our heart energy, our passion, purpose, desires, wants, and dreams. In addition, we are balancing this with our head energy, cultural programming, what we believe we can achieve, our thoughts of accomplishing our dreams, rationalizations, and following unspoken and spoken rules (family, work, church, society).

When I brought these possibilities to her attention, she immediately knew what this pain related to in her life. She didn't feel comfortable expressing it out loud, so I told her to just relax and allow herself to let go of her suppression of her true expression. I encouraged her to allow herself to imagine seeing, doing, having, and being the exact person, she envisioned herself to be. I reminded her that neck pain is related to life issues around "sticking your neck out" often for others rather than yourself. It also is about being inflexible in your attitudes and beliefs or in dealing with people, things, or situations in your life. All of this stuck energy was showing up in physical form since she was having difficulty turning her head to the left and it was painful when she did. I shared she was showing blocks that indicated she was holding onto and burying things from her past. I told her that if the pain and stiffness were more right-sided then this would indicate that she is experiencing fear about looking into her future.

Flexibility is about being able to adapt to the variety of situations that may arise at any given moment. Most of the time we are incredibly flexible beings. However, if we are in a state of being overwhelmed, then our flexibility or ability to move in our lives becomes more limited. When we are under stressful situations or experience stress from our emotions, we often feel like we need to fight, take flight, or freeze. This leaves you feeling like you have limited choices in life. Then, of the choices you do have, you may feel like you are not empowered with a voice to express yourself. The result often is you wake up with a stiff neck. You can't turn your head to see all the possibilities that are around you. Did you stay with me on that?

If there is something in your present life that stimulates a memory or an energy pattern from your past that you have chosen not to process, you may indeed wake up one morning with a neck so stiff you can't turn your head to the left. I see and hear this so many times in my office. "Doc, I woke up this morning and just couldn't turn my head." "Oh," is my typical response. "Which side is most difficult to turn to?" "My left," is the reply. Your body says, in no uncertain terms, that there is an issue from your past that you are not willing to look at completely. You may say to me as an astute student of body insights and the Health Code that there could be something in the patient's past that has caused them to literally freeze when it comes to moving forward. They may have halted taking an action step to move forward in their life. Alternatively, for instance, if a person can't bend their head forward then the body-mind is saying, "There is something right in front of your face that you are unwilling to see or where you are just being totally inflexible." If you can't bend your head back, then there may be something from the past that is creating a pattern of inflexibility. There may be a trigger stimulating you in the present that is causing you pain and stiffness. And the right side indicates pain about future momentum. It all ends up coming together in some way or the body wouldn't be sending out that particular message. If the body-mind had a different message, it would choose some other place to express pain or discomfort.

Continuing with a different neck ailment, the upper cervical area, the area just below the skull, is interesting to consider from an emotional standpoint. It is the area where the brain and the nervous system connect, the anatomical connection of the body-mind interplay. This is where the dancing impulses of the neurons lead to the manifestation of physiology and where ideas, thoughts, dreams, and "Aha's!" become material stuff of the Universe. Deepak Chopra, M.D., a renowned endocrinologist and thought leader of the body-mind movement, says in his book, *Perfect Health*, "Every time there is an event in the mind, there is a corresponding event in the body. All your hopes, fears, dreams, and wishes, along with the faintest wisps of emotion and desire, have left their marks on your physiology—these mental events constantly shape the body as they 'talk' to it."

I first understood that the memory of any given situation or circumstance is remembered not only in the mind but in the body as well when I was working with clients who had been injured in automobile accidents. Though the injuries would resolve, months later they would show up in my office again, complaining of the exact same symptoms as before. I would discover that they had not been in another accident but had been sitting at a stoplight on a rainy night; they had heard the screeching of tires but had not been struck by another vehicle. Every time there is an event in the mind, there is a corresponding event in the body. The body remembers, especially if the event is similar enough to an earlier event that resulted in trauma to the body. The resolution of this process, I discovered, was to heal the body, and also heal, erase, or desensitize the body to the emotions and memory of the original event.

When a person has pain at the very top of the spine, specifically called the upper cervical area, this gives us a clue that they are having a very difficult time integrating their thoughts and ideas into action. It may be a problem with integrating some aspect of their spiritual life or their desire for a spiritual connectedness into their daily lifestyle. The entire neck, but specifically the upper cervical area, is where the head and the heart either connect or conflict. The neck is an energy conduit between the heart (your passions and desire) and your head (your cultural programming and societal scripting). It is, in other words, where you have been letting your head run your life and have not given your heart its part in the decision-making process. You have a certain "mind set" and you have forgotten your "heart set." Following the lead of your heart is probably one of the most difficult things to learn and at the same time is one of the most important and life-changing things you can do. Your heart's path is the path of truth.

The Upper Arm, Strictly Humerus, Ha! Ha!

From the standpoint of the emotional gateways and looking at the extremities, the upper arm represents the Expression Gateway. The upper arm is connected to the shoulder. In human anatomy, it is commonly called the humerus. The humerus is the name of the bone found in the upper arm. As far as I'm concerned, it is actually not too far off in its name. Pain or stiffness in the upper arm is truly related to your loss of humor. It's about where you have allowed life to become too serious; the humor of day to day life is lost or gone. Humor, as an expression, is vital to our immune system and to our ability to adapt to the challenges that life presents along our journey. If we are unable to find the fun, laughter, and humor along the way then it is our own chosen perspective on things that is most likely getting in our way. As a driver in Ireland told me, "Ireland is like life—if you aren't having fun in Ireland it's your own fault". Pain in the upper arm is about the loss of humor in your life. It's about not seeing life as a comedy, and the funny thing is, it is all a comedy.

Sometimes we feel that we are the brunt of the joke. Sometimes we feel like we are the joke. Sometimes everyone is laughing except us. Bummer way to feel, don't you think? One thing, among many, I learned through my cancer treatment is that life and the things that make us stuck are all a joke. When all is said and done, all this stuff we take so intensely isn't going to matter one little bit when we are done with this life. Many of us are at a place where we take life too seriously. If we could just cultivate the ability to laugh at ourselves more and criticize ourselves less, we would develop a whole new relationship with stress in our lives. Give it up! Find the humor. Fill every day (at least each week) of your life with just a little bit of humor, a light-hearted joke, see a crazy, funny movie (rather than one of the multitudes of violent ones) or sit with your family or friends and tell humorous tales from our past.

The Thigh or Upper Leg

The Expression Gateway in the lower extremity is the upper leg or thigh. This area of the leg has most to do with stepping out or moving forward in your life. We all have experienced an inner urge that arises for us, some of us more than others, to move forward or change direction, to "step out there." This can be changing jobs or careers, about investing money, time, or energy in a specific project, or trying something new like a language, dating, skydiving, or a creative endeavor. There is a part of us that is totally excited about the newness of the adventure and another part of us that is petrified, mortified, or at least paralyzed by fear. Anyone ever been there? I know I have. This particular gateway in this area of the body is associated with that balance between expression and suppression. It's about speaking out, having a voice, and expressing your truth. Many of us get caught in the other side of this where we continue to try to please others instead of taking care of ourselves and our movement forward.

My client, Willie, came to me complaining of hip and thigh pain that he couldn't quite explain as far as an injury history. He owned a furniture business and thought maybe he had pulled a muscle or strained himself lifting or moving some furniture. On closer examination and questioning, as well as breathing and bringing his body awareness to his thigh pain, he was able to open to the bio-emotional messages. His current career and job stress arose, which was a surprise to both of us. He told me that he was in the process of selling his furniture business. He also stated that he was uncertain as to the next step he was going to take to feel inspired to express himself in a creative way. After clearing many emotions that were limiting his decision-making process, we then worked to discover what his desired creative expression might be. It turned out to be painting! So, we identified his subconscious beliefs about work and play or work versus play.

We worked with his belief about it being okay to fully express himself for the pure desire of expressing creatively. I gave him a homework assignment to follow for the next 30 days. I told him he had to paint every day for those 30 days and then come back and see if there was more work to be done around his beliefs and perceptions. Willie returned a month later and stated that he had finished a minimum of 18 paintings and was in love with his new way of being in the world. He ultimately sold his furniture business and took on painting full-time in his "retirement." To this day, he teaches and holds gallery openings for many of his paintings. He is in love with his new creative expression and enjoying his full-time painting career.

So, sometimes this frustration with our future will appear in the form of thigh or leg pain, strain, or discomfort. What is metaphorically happening is that the front of the leg is trying to move forward while the back of the thigh, the hamstring, is desperately holding back with all its might. The oh-so-common hamstring pull that debilitates many a track star before a contest can often be understood from this emotional point of view. The injury can be attributed to the intense emotional struggle between the competitive part of the athlete's mind wanting to be the first, best, and fastest, and the self-doubting part pulling back so as not to look bad if the athlete loses or fails. Can you begin to see how these unnecessary inner struggles, if not handled, accepted, or processed can manifest in big, physical ways to attract our attention?

Thyroid

Here is another example of where two organ systems, thyroid and adrenals, in the acupuncture meridian system are closely related in their physiological function. It has been long known that if you are suffering from hypothyroidism (lowered function of the thyroid gland) then you are already suffering adrenal stress in your body.

Although the thyroid gland is associated with the Expression Gateway and the adrenal gland is associated with the Foundation Gateway (root chakra), this is where the acupuncture system and the hormonal system collaborate in the communication between these coupled meridians. In the acupuncture system, these organs are linked together. Remember that the Expression Gateway is about the expression of yourself—your truth, purpose in life, and creativity. The Expression Gateway's emphasis is projecting your unique creativity into the world. It is easy to see how the thyroid and its emotions of expression verse suppression, coupled with the adrenal gland being about having the flexibility to be yourself expressed in the world, could easily support or conflict with each other. The conflict of blocked emotions or suppressed expression could easily happen for most of us.

Emotions that are associated uniquely with the thyroid gland are muddled instability, muddled thinking, emotional instability, and paranoia. Muddled instability is when things feel mucked up, confused, messy, and unstable all at the same time. Paranoia in this particular case is the fearful victimization that many people feel from just being in life every day. Since the thyroid is part of the Expression Gateway, often these emotions that we just listed come from our own self-suppression or from a cultural suppression that exists. We often learn to not speak out of turn, to hold back our unique gifts and talents from the world. Many of us get confused about our true purpose and path and this gets in the way of making appropriate decisions to move forward in our lives. Since this lack of motivation tends to keep us stagnant in our progress by default, we then naturally suppress our expression in the world.

Some of the other thyroid blocked emotions are pretty self-explanatory. With these emotions, I often see patients with those "up and down" feelings that we experience, as well as the "I can't figure it out" feelings. As a matter of fact, I often will hear these exact words come out of the patient's mouth. They will say something like, "I just can't figure out what I need to do in this particular case." Bingo! I immediately start checking their energy around the thyroid or adrenals. When I find the best way to support their adrenal/thyroid system, they will often come in just days later and state that it became so clear what they needed to do to resolve their previous problem.

Awareness Keys

- The Expression Gateway is all about communication, verbal or non-verbal, created from internal or external. It's about creatively turning ideas into reality.

- Blocks in the Expression Gateway can show as not being able to keep secrets, telling lies or feeling a lack of connection with your vocation or purpose in life.

- The neck is an energy conduit between the heart and the head. Pay attention to where your heart's desires are being ruled by that overly rational head of yours.

- The upper arm, just below the shoulder, is about your loss of humor. Ask yourself: where am I being too serious or taking life too seriously?

- Fill each day or at least each week of your life with a little bit of humor.

- The thigh or upper leg is about moving forward in your life. It's about speaking out and expressing your truth.

- Many of us get blocked trying to please others instead of taking care of ourselves.

- The thigh is where the push / pull of moving forward in your life is in direct conflict with your self-doubt holding you back.

- The thyroid is about when things feel mucked up, confused, messy or unstable. Or we are just playing that old familiar tune of fearful victimization.

- The thyroid is also that organ that stores those feelings of "I can't figure it out" or the emotions of the oh-so-typical "ups and downs" of life.

Chapter 8

The Love Gateway

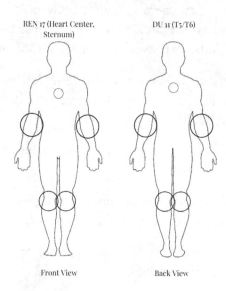

REN 17 (Heart Center, Sternum)

DU 11 (T5/T6)

Front View

Back View

This gateway is aligned with the heart chakra at the center of the chest through to the thoracic spine. Its color is green. This gateway fills our life with compassion, love, and beauty. It is driven by the principles of transformation and integration. This gateway also creates the bridge between earthly and spiritual aspirations. The love gateway, heart center, also includes the thymus gland, which is our main organ of regulating the immune system and its health and wellness.

The main meaning or functions associated with the Love Gateway are love for oneself and others, relationships, compassion, and forgiveness. It is associated with empathy, acceptance, change, and transformation. It assists us and helps process grieving and in finding peace and discernment, in addition to integration of insights. It is our center of awareness. The most common feelings of an open Love Gateway are a sense of connectedness, a harmonious exchange of energy with all that is around you, and an appreciation of natural beauty.

If there is imbalance in the Love Gateway, you may experience difficulty relating to others, excessive jealousy, codependency, being closed down or withdrawn. It is the connection between lower gateways or energy centers and upper gateways or energy centers. This gateway acts as a center of integration of earthly matters and higher aspirations. It integrates the balance of these two energies effortlessly and harmoniously.

When imbalanced, these things may manifest: being overly defensive, feeling closed down, and a fear of intimacy. It manifests as codependency by relying on other's approval and attention, being a pleaser at all cost, putting oneself in the role of rescuer or falling into victim mode. It will exhibit as being reclusive, isolating oneself, being or feeling antisocial. It will also manifest in not forgiving or holding grudges.

Thymus Gland

The thymus is the main organ of the immune system. It is located in the center of the chest just below the sternum. It is associated with the Love Gateway/heart chakra, and emotionally is where we process the emotions of resignation and the feelings of resigning oneself. It is where we carry our feelings of being troubled, attacked, or where we feel overwhelmed or perhaps attacking others. Since the Love Gateway is about love, joy, and inner peace, you can see how it might be easy to have the thymus gland affected by our broken loves, disappointments, and chaos. Our lives are often filled with opportunities to feel overwhelmed and troubled not only in our personal experiences, but also by the world around us. We can get affected by the conflict in our culture—between our desire to feel connected and to experience a harmony of energies with others versus how great the disconnect in our culture currently is. When we don't get the connection we are seeking, which unfortunately for most people is the case, our thymus has to store this sense of emotional overload. This may very well be why most people are more and more susceptible to disease processes. Their immune systems are already emotionally overwhelmed. Then, considering that we have more virulent bacteria and virus outbreaks, we just don't have the immune stamina to resist them.

In my own story, the thymus played an essential role in my disease process. If you remember the story, I had returned from Panama with a renewed commitment to make my practice and my life different than how it had been in my previous practice experience. Yet, I returned to my old habits and over the three years following my return, I was back in my old patterns. It was then that I began to resign myself to the reality that I might not ever change my ways, even though I had all of the intention to do so. That not only left me feeling helpless, but also left me feeling overwhelmed by the fact that I didn't think I had it in me to make the change. This emotional stress certainly played a critical role in my compromised immune system and left the door wide open to the possibility of cancer or other diseases.

Heart

If you have noticed in previous discussion, the coupled meridians from the acupuncture system share neighboring chakras that are known to share energy with one another. My friends and mentors, Karen Curry Parker and Michelle Vandepas, expand this approach to better understanding ourselves through Human Design. We often see that in the complexity of emotions that we experience, the mix of emotions is often shared by neighboring chakras and meridians as well. With this in mind, the heart and small mix of emotions is energetically linked together in the acupuncture system and neurologically through the vagus nerve systems. The small intestine is an organ of digestion though is associated with the Action Gateway (solar plexus chakra) while the heart is associated with the Love Gateway (heart chakra).

Neurologically, both the heart and the small intestine organs are linked by the vagus nerve. This nerve is well known in emotional trauma literature for its influence in the body-mind communication. That may be why when you get your heart broken, you feel like "doo-doo". Just kidding. (However, this may not be so far off after all.) In taking a closer look, the heart is associated with the emotions of connection, love for oneself and others, compassion, and forgiveness. If you look at the Organ Systems and Emotions Chart included in the next section, you will see that there are many emotions associated with heart issues and how we digest (ha, nice pun) our experiences in life. One of my favorite emotions to use is "frightfully overjoyed." You are probably asking, "what the heck is 'frightfully overjoyed' anyway? Have you ever been in a situation where you were really anticipating some event and joyfully excited about it, yet, at the same time scared to death? That's the feeling.

Take a common experience like marriage. You're excited; maybe it's something you know you want to do. The person you are marrying brings a lot of joy to your life and you are actually excited about spending the rest of your life with them. When it comes to the wedding itself, you are thinking about a bunch of people watching you, the things you need to remember to do and say, and so, your nerves start rattling just thinking about the day of the wedding. That is the combination of joy and fright or fear overlapping with each other and often you can't separate the feelings. This confusion causes much distress for many couples and often creates heartburn or worse. When the coupled meridian goes into action, this may lead to the intestinal symptom of diarrhea just before the fateful day. You may have experienced this body-mind interaction or at least know someone who has.

Current science research, specifically from the Heart Math Institute, has discovered that the heart and small intestine are rich in neurological activity. As I mentioned earlier in this section, the neurology of the body-mind connection to both the heart and the small intestine is heavily documented and studied. The heart continues to help us integrate our earthly motivations and personal aspirations with the higher aspiration of altruism and our spiritual nature. When we are unbalanced in the heart, we may find ourselves closed down, withdrawn, or not being able to relate to others as well. Remember that the antithesis of living life with an open, expressive Love Gateway is living in fear.

Lung

In the same-partnered manner, the lung and large intestines are also coupled meridians in the acupuncture system and in the Health Code system. These two share a number of emotions together and yet have their individual areas of uniqueness. The lung is part of the Love Gateway and the large intestines are part of the Pleasure Gateway. The lung shares many of the same emotions as the large intestine; however, the lung is most commonly associated with the emotions of grief, anguish, yearning, and sadness.

Susan presented to my office with what appeared to be a respiratory infection. It was evident by her chest congestion, cough, and raspy voice. On asking about her symptoms, she stated that she had neither had the flu or a cold, nor had she been exposed to anyone that was contagious with an illness. On further questioning, it became apparent that this had surfaced following the death of her mother and the realization that this was her last parent to die. She was feeling a deep sense of loss, grief, and aloneness. I can't tell you how many times someone has lost a loved one and developed an upper respiratory infection or respiratory distress immediately following the event. I was able to help Susan move through the grief process much quicker and within a few days she was feeling normal again, without the signs or symptoms of respiratory distress.

When you are anguishing over the anticipation of something or anguishing over something that happened in the past that you wish you could change, the lung and large intestines have to process this. When you have a yearning to make something different, or for something to be different, often times this energy disturbance will also end up as a symptom in these systems too.

Mid-Back: Thoracic Spine

The thoracic spine is the next area of focus as we move through the gateways of the body, and specifically the spinal column. The thoracic spine is a large biogeographical area, encompassing the majority of the spine. In Eastern medicine, for example, medical approaches like acupuncture, Jin Shin, Tai Chi, and other practices associate areas of the body with specific organ systems. In

Western medicine, many organ systems refer pain to specific areas of the body. For instance, kidney dysfunction often refers pain to the low back; heart dysfunction to the arm, shoulder, and chest. The area often found painful in patients is the area between the shoulder blades, referred to as the mid-back area. This area is most often associated with the organ systems of liver and gall bladder on the right side of the area between the shoulder blades. On the left side between the shoulder blades, it is associated with the pancreas and spleen. Even though most of these organs are associated with the Action Gateway, we will cover them here because of their relationship to the thoracic spine.

This is the longest section of the spinal column and the thoracic spinal nerves innervate most of the organs of both the Action and Love Gateways. When there is an overlap of gateways and organ systems confusion can ensue. I'm hoping that this overlap might just help you understand more deeply how multiple emotions can make a greater pattern of energy disharmony. For example, the liver is most often associated with the emotions of anger, resentment, frustration, or irritation. Other emotions that are associated with this area from the pancreas and spleen are feelings of low self-esteem and self-criticism. These are all organs of the Action Gateway. Issues of the heart are also associated with this spinal area and are usually found slightly higher. The heart area is in the upper back between the shoulder blades and up to the lower neck. Emotions that are related to the heart are feeling lost, vulnerable, abandoned, deserted, or insecure. The upper thoracic spine is associated with the heart chakra and the Love Gateway; it's the seat of all emotion, your truth. You can easily see how you could experience liver and gall bladder emotions of anger, resentment, frustration or irritation in addition to heart emotions of feeling lost, vulnerable, abandoned, or deserted. The mid to lower thoracic spine is associated with the Action Gateway and solar plexus chakra, which is the seat of your personal power, identity, will, and clarity of judgment. Again, you can see how the pancreas and spleen emotions of self-doubt and being self-critical could easily be a response to feelings of lack of personal power, identity, and personal will. I may have beat this drum a bit too hard, but my point is, that emotions are complex, not just simply one thing or the other. Our emotions get laid down in layers during an event and sometimes it is a process of unraveling that complexity.

The thoracic spine has two transition areas. The upper area of transition is where the neck and shoulders meet. The lower area of transition is the small of the back or the kidney area. When these areas are involved in the symptom picture, you might get the insight to consider where you are making a painful or un-comfortable transition in your life. Let's say, for instance, you are leaving a relationship. The transition of leaving the relationship and moving into a new lifestyle could create pain in either of the transition zones of the thoracic spine. If you were feeling resent-ment in the transition, you might experience upper thoracic pain, resentment being more of a liver emotion or heart emotion. If you are feeling unsupported in this transition, more of a low back emotion, then you will experience lower thoracic pain.

Bella, for example, is a young high school graduate who is moving to college. She is an athlete and she was experiencing lower back pain with tension. She has been lovingly supported by her mother and her extended family. Her athletic ability is one of the means by which she will be able to afford her college tui-tion through athletic scholarships, grants, and loans. She is expe-riencing fear that she will not be able to balance the demands of her school schedule and maintain her position on the team. She is also feeling the financial tension that she can't afford school if she doesn't perform both in athletics as well as academically. She is feeling stress about not letting her family down. She is conflicted in her foundation by feeling she has to balance family and the finances of school. Not to mention the fears of change that come with this next stage of life. Oh, did I mention that her boyfriend of six years is a junior in high school, so she will also be leaving him behind? Ouch!! Tell me that doesn't create some sympathetic low back pain for you just hearing this story.

Here is the rest of the story. She resolved the issues within herself of letting the family down, no matter what she does. She became aware that her family is the village that has always had her back. No pun intended. Through our work, she knows un-doubtedly that she is supported in her life in whatever makes her shine. She not only will get scholarships for her academics and athletics, but she has a job with the college as well. She now understands that she has a secondary support system, the college staff and teachers who want her to be successful in completing her degree program. Her pain moved for a temporary amount of time to the region of her back called the thoraco-lumbar region. (As mentioned above, this is represented by a spinal transition zone as well as a zone of transition in life.) Her stress? The boyfriend. She is now resolved that, even though they are crazy in love, she is learning to take care of herself and her future. If he is respectful enough to support her in this transition, then they will have a great chance at making a go of their relationship for the long term. If not, she is getting some valuable information for the future of this relationship. Currently, she is doing well. As an aside, her athletics, college, family, and boyfriend are also all doing well. She has relaxed into the clarity she is experiencing. She is pain and tension free after releasing the energy blockages held in thoracic region.

The Ribs

Intimately associated with the thoracic spine and the Love Gateway is, of course, the rib cage, which protects the heart. During the phases of respiration—inhalation and expiration—the ribs expand and contract, move up and down. We know that the sternum (breast bone) that connects the ribs on the front of the body will actually tighten the ligament attachments to protect the heart from metaphoric injury. This typically will happen after trauma or loss. Our egos get involved and by default declare our heart incapable of handling the loss. (They will break after all, you know.) But really the heart and its chakra are about our capacity to love; it is the home of our emotional processing. From what you've learned so far, what insights do you think the ribs have to do with in the body? You got it! It's being able to "take in" or "receive" in your life, and to "let go of," or "give away," in life. Throughout our lives we are inhaling the experiences of our lives. Ideally, we are integrating these experiences, getting our lessons, and then letting go of what we can't use or don't need to hang onto any longer. When you have rib pain or feel constricted when taking a breath, you may want to examine how well you are able to take in the experiences that are occurring in your life. There may be something that has happened that you are really having a difficult time processing. Maybe you are resisting something that doesn't fit your value system. Like Bella and her values about putting her own life in front of the needs of everyone else. It is terribly painful to realize this incongruence in your value system, and sometimes even more difficult to incorporate that realization with the appropriate action steps and congruent behaviors into your life.

Conversely, if you experience more pain on exhalation, then you may want to examine your inability to let go of some painful event in your life. The rib cage surrounds and encompasses the lungs, which we now know have most to do with grief and sadness. The rib cage is potentially a treasure chest of shared emotions because it surrounds the lungs, thymus, and heart. However, if you have lost a loved one or are carrying grief over a disappointment in your life, you may be unable to let go of the disappointment or sadness. You may subconsciously be holding onto a part of your breath that contains this sadness, grief, or disappointment. That constant grip will cause a painful rigidity in the muscles surrounding the spine and ribs.

The Elbow

The Elbow is about your ability to be emotionally flexible. Can you bend, or be bendable, in your approach to a situation or circumstance that appears in your life? Can you be flexible if a challenge or situation is presented to you from someone else? Are you bending too much, like bending over backward to accommodate someone else's needs versus maintaining your own boundaries? Are you bending out of your comfort zone so far that you are vulnerable or at risk to your own good? These are standard Love Gateway emotions. You will find in the next story the theme of the Love Gateway of feeling connected to your purpose, relationship to others, and feeling a harmonious exchange of energy with all that is around you.

My friend and client, Bobby, came to me for elbow pain in both his left and right arms. Bobby has known me a long time and is very familiar with my approach to body-mind healing. He came to me wanting to discover what underlying emotions might be aggravating his bilateral elbow challenge. With a thorough evaluation and no direct physical cause other than inflammation being found, we explored the possible emotions that were directly affecting his pain. The left side metaphorically representing the past led us to discover that he was bending over backward to support his family. He had at the time one child of an adult age still living at home, who was not working to bring in income to help with the family. His wife was also not working to help with income. She was mostly relaxing at home, talking about working, but actually not contributing to the ongoing financial burdens of the household. Now, Bobby was not one to complain and he was happy to sacrifice his own time and energy to support his family. However, his body was shouting at him in the form of elbow pain. The question became does he want to continue this pattern or evolve past it? He decided that he would continue in this pattern. So we worked together to release his inner burden feeling with this conscious decision. With the release of the energy and a new perspective, his left elbow pain shifted.

We then explored his right elbow pain. We uncovered that the work he was doing with his employer was just too rigid of a job. He was not expressing his true purpose, passion, and nature through his approach to his work. What the company needed and actually had hired him to do was to be more of a spiritual anchor for the company as a whole. Since he was not able to fulfill his role due to other demands on his time and energy, the company was flailing around somewhat unsuccessful. I asked him if he could step into his true role with the company. A light of inspiration and realization went off in his body-mind. He said resoundingly "Yes, I can!" He knew exactly how he needed to show up for himself, honor his true nature, and benefit the company. He took action by changing his mindset and behavior and almost immediately the company excelled and grew. The side story is that both left and right elbow pain went away initially. However, the left elbow pain had not completely resolved, even though the pain went away. A year later, he almost died from an aortic aneurysm. His heart was about to explode. From a body insight and Health Code way of thinking, I believe the situation at home was breaking his heart and he felt he couldn't change it. Sometimes we can choose to behave in ways that are too generous with our love and energy. Not that this is a bad behavior. But, if we can't openly talk about it, or when we realize it we don't change our behavior, it might be creating personal damage. This conflict or stuck energy may be putting our health at risk.

You see, elbows are associated with the heart, the Love Gateway and also related to unconditional love issues. Unconditional love is often about generosity in your life. This generosity is not necessarily monetarily, but more about a persistent energy pattern of not being open-hearted with sharing yourself. It may show up in you not being real with people, not acting in integrity with yourself and others, and not sharing your feelings. We call this not being generous with your gifts, talents, and abilities in the world. Affectionately, we refer to it as being stingy. You could choose to ask yourself if you are being stingy, stiff, or inflexible about forgiving someone. Are you being generous enough as a human being to allow the other person to just be unconditionally loved by you? Maybe this isn't about someone else, but in reality, this is about treating yourself in this way?

Let go and just be okay with who you are, stop being so hard on yourself. You can stop your own suffering anytime you want. You just have to make the choice to stop. Love is the answer; love is the way. Suffering, whether we see it or not, or for that matter like it or not, is self-imposed. Suffering is an inside job. You are the only one who can do it to yourself and you are the only one who is allowing it to continue. You are the only one who can stop it as well.

The Knee

Now, the knee, much like the elbow, is about flexibility and a person's ability to bend to a situation or circumstance. The knee, however, is often associated with not bending enough or bending too much to allow you to move forward. It incorporates the issues we already discussed about the inner struggles. Do I give too much? Am I not giving enough love and support? Again, Love Gateway emotions associated with the Love Gateway and heart chakra are all colored with love and compassion for self and others. What is often important in healing knee pain is unconditionally loving yourself while resolving the physical dysfunction in the knee. The knee, unlike the elbow, often incorporates the concept of support or feeling unsupported in these issues. In addition to the knee is the knee cap or patella, and one often may experience deep knee pain or pain deep in the joint. It is often discovered through the Health Code exploration that a person may be hiding some deeply held belief or self-criticism. This self-criticism then may not be fully apparent because it is being covered or hidden by some other behavior. If you are suffering from arthritis of the knee, I would question whether there is something that is literally "eating away at you." A situation or experience that is limiting your ability to unconditionally love yourself or someone else. The condition, arthritis, anywhere in the body is metaphoric for "something or someone eating away at you."

Awareness Keys

- The Love Gateway is about compassion, love, and beauty, and drives our transformation and integration of all energy.

- The Love Gateway is also associated with the thymus gland and regulates our immune system.

- The Love Gateway is about love of self and others, relationships, and forgiveness. It is associated with empathy, acceptance, and change. It is most importantly about connectedness.

- The Love Gateway acts as a center of integration between earthly matters and your higher altruistic aspirations. When the Love Gateway is closed down you may experience difficulty relating to others. You may feel closed down, withdrawn, defensive. You may experience fear of intimacy or codependency.

- The thymus gland is where we harbor resignation, feelings of being troubled or attacked.

- The thymus gland being in the Love Gateway is easily affected by our broken loves, disappointment and the current global "disconnect" between people.

- The heart and small intestine are shared meridians and neurologically connected to the vagus nerve.

- In trauma psychology, the polyvagal theory makes the connection of the brain, emotional heart and the small intestines through the vagus nerve.

- Ultimately you either live your life with an open Love Gateway experience or live in fear.

- The lung is part of the Love Gateway and is associated with grief, anguish, yearning and sadness.

- The thoracic spine has many overlapping areas and gateways, Love and Action Gateways specifically.

- The mid-thoracic area to the lower neck area is mostly associated with the heart, liver and gallbladder organs.

- The area between the shoulder blades is associated with the heart, liver, pancreas and spleen organs.

- The thoracic spine has two transition areas. Upper, between the cervical and thoracic spine and lower, between the thoracic spine and the low back. These are involved with the emotions of transition in any form as well.

- The ribs and the Love Gateway are about protection of the heart.

- Ribs represent our ability to "take in" or "receive" in life and "give away" or "let goof" in life.

- The elbow is about your ability to be emotionally flexible.

- Elbows are associated with the Love Gateway and being generous with your gifts, talents, and abilities, or about being "stingy".

- The knee like the elbow is also about flexibility and our ability to bend to a situation or circumstance. However, the knee is more about unconditional love for yourself and feeling supported in the process.

Chapter 9

The Action Gateway

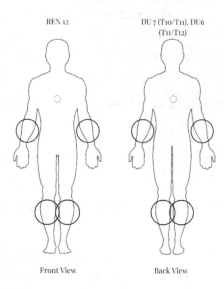

REN 12   DU 7 (T10/T11), DU6
                              (T11/T12)

Front View   Back View

The next area of our focus is the Action Gateway, which aligns with the solar plexus chakra, the stomach area. Its color is yellow. This center is about radiating your personal power in the world. It is about the expression of will, mental abilities, and asserting your uniqueness in the world. It is associated with taking responsibility for one's life, forming personal opinions and beliefs, and making decisions. It is exhibited through setting our direction for action and clarity of judgment. It manifests in our personal identity, our self-assurance and self-discipline, and our independence.

This center gives us the actual momentum to move forward and realize our personal desires as well as intentions in the world. It gives us the actions to take in order to reach our goals. Imbalances that are associated with the Action Gateway are undermining our self-esteem and social life. These issues can manifest as excessive control over our environment and people. It can be deficient or blocked, creating feelings of helplessness, irresponsibility, or being obsessed with minute details. We will see life through a filter of plus and minuses while losing sight of the whole picture. It can manifest as being manipulative and misusing your power. It could also manifest as a lack of clear direction, lack of purpose or ambition, difficulty, or the lack of making plans. Often it exhibits by having lots of ideas, but not finding a way to realize them.

Small Intestine

As we shared in the section on the heart, the small intestine shares a neurological connection with the heart via the vagus nerve and is also a linked meridian in the acupuncture system with the heart meridian. The small intestine, however, is more associated with the feelings of vulnerability, abandonment, and the emotion of feeling like you are lost. Not like you are lost in your neighborhood and can't find your way home. More the feeling of being lost about what to do in a situation or lost as to what is the appropriate action to take in a circumstance. It is associated with the feeling of being deserted or abandoned as well, which often leaves us with feelings of insecurity.

Since the small intestine is associated with the Action Gateway, you can see how the above feelings might stand in the way of the positive aspect of action. These feelings can and do sidetrack us from realizing our personal desires, and taking the action needed to reach our goals. The unbalanced expression of the small intestine could show up for us as lack of purpose or feelings of helplessness. The culture in which we live creates way too many small intestine dysfunctions, from food sensitivities to ulcers. These symptoms are expressions of our lack of clear direction, the expression of our will, taking responsibility for our life, and also the stress of just making decisions.

Stomach, Spleen, and Pancreas

The stomach, spleen, and pancreas are all organs found below the diaphragm and are coupled acupuncture meridian systems. The spleen in Chinese medicine is responsible for the task of both the pancreas and spleen, as we know them in Western science. The roles attributed to the spleen organ truly encompass both the pancreas' and the spleen's activities in our body. These three organs have similar emotions and give us insights that are often tied in with each other. The Action Gateway is associated with both the stomach and pancreas, mostly because they are organs of digestion.

We most often think of the stomach in the Health Code as having to do with the feelings of disgust or of being overly sympathetic. Overly sympathetic is expressed in two ways, as either feeling sorry for another or feeling sorry for one's self. So, if you are having stomach problems, dysfunction, or pain, it could be that you are feeling sorry for someone else or it may be a situation where you are having a pity party for yourself.

When confronted with pancreas problems, such as low or high blood sugar, diabetes, or even digestive enzyme dysfunction, we think of self-criticism or self-doubt. These aren't the only emotions that could be harbored in the pancreas tissue, but are the ones most often associated if you are experiencing mood swings, sugar cravings or maybe gas and bloating after eating. Using the Health Code, you might inquire into where you are having self-doubt or second thoughts about something. Maybe you should just lighten up on yourself about those things for which you are hammering (criticizing) yourself. Or better yet, just love yourself for who you are, stop the criticism, and realize you are okay just as you are. Forgiveness!

Adrenals

The adrenal glands are associated with the Action Gateway. The adrenal glands are about radiating your personal power. They support personal expansion and the formation of identity through relating to others and the world. They are characterized by movement and flow in our emotions and thoughts. The emotional aspect of the adrenals is so well known that we just take the description as normal. It is about emotional exhaustion, running on empty, and being drained of our life force. Most of the overload for clients is dealing with feelings of over-responsibility and not being able to carry that load any longer.

Many people in our society are suffering from weak or low-functioning adrenal glands. Adrenals are our flight, fight, or freeze response organs and they respond readily to stress in our lives. For many of us, just waking up to face the morning is stressful and then it just goes downhill from there. In the last few years, I have seen an incredible increase in the number of clients who are experiencing adrenal fatigue coinciding with low thyroid function. Common symptoms of this are fatigue, weight gain, foggy headed feeling, low sex drive, and depression.

The current theory on low thyroid function associated with adrenal fatigue is explained like this: The adrenal glands, being our first line of defense in managing our daily stress, eventually can no longer carry on the task adequately and so become exhausted. At this point the stressors don't necessarily stop, so the adrenal glands begin the process of borrowing energy from the thyroid gland. The thyroid being the manager of our metabolism grows tired of trying to prop-up the energy of the body in handling our daily stress levels. You might have noticed that our daily stress levels have gotten much more intense over the years. Eventually the thyroid can't handle it anymore and it begins to decrease its function. As a last resort, the body then starts to borrow energy from the sex organs, which then puts our overall energy level in the basement

Liver

The liver and gallbladder actually work together in their physiological relationship, and together energetically, as coupled meridians. The liver is most classically associated with emotions of anger, resentment, irritation, and frustration. In my practice, I most often see it being related to anger and frustration. It is part of the Action Gateway and therefore associated with the exertion of our will and asserting ourselves in the world. As an unbalanced excess of energy, it can exhibit as excessive control over our environment and people. It will show up as manipulative or misuse of our power and specifically anger. There have actually been studies done on people experiencing anger situations and then testing their levels of liver enzymes. Many of these levels were elevated immediately following these incidences. A deficiency of energy, the emotion of depression, is associated with the liver as well. This is a great place to discuss the concept that emotional states affect the physiological function of the organ itself. One thing most people don't realize, though, is that physiological dysfunction in an organ system can also affect the emotions a person will experience. So, in a nutshell, if you are an alcoholic, which is known to destroy liver cells and cause cellular dysfunction within the liver, you will more than likely experience anger and depression as predominant emotions. On the other side of this debate, if you are experiencing lots of anger and depression in your life, you very well may develop serious liver dysfunction, abnormal liver enzymes, or even chronic liver disease.

Gallbladder

The gallbladder is energetically and physiologically associated with the liver in that it stores bile from the liver. The bile is then used to assist in digestion in the small intestines. The gallbladder is associated with the emotions of dread, resentment, and feeling embittered and soured on life. People with gallbladder dysfunction are intensely irritated with other people and the world around them. A client may be lacking the guts to take decisive corrective action around a situation. As the gallbladder is part of the Action Gateway this makes perfect sense. They often are convinced that they are the only ones capable of making the right decisions, choices, and judgments. When imbalanced, the emotions of the gallbladder can manifest as greed, willfulness, power addiction, and self-centered anger.

Since the gallbladder is a sac that is attached by a small tube to the liver, it is not a large stretch of the imagination to think about anger that drains from the liver into the holding bin of the gallbladder. Like most unresolved anger, if allowed to sit or get stagnant, it could become resentment (a gallbladder emotion). If resentment is left long enough unresolved or unexpressed, like most attitudes, it might become hardened (kind of like a gallstone) and ultimately cause us a great deal of pain. Gallstones may very well be the result of a long held unresolved anger that has turned into a deep resentment.

The Forearm

In the Health Code, the forearm is part of the Action Gateway of the upper extremity. The forearm emotions are about control, both trying to control or take control. In controlling, we are either controlling from our past experience or trying to control our future experience. Remember back to our thoughts on where the past versus the future might show up in the body. Trying to control the past would most likely exhibit symptoms in the left forearm. Whereas, trying to control our future most likely would express symptoms in the right forearm. This appears in so many ways that they are too numerous to list. The point is that you can't control much of anything in life because in reality there is nothing to control. Life is what it is. If you are trying to control something, you are either living from your past or living into a predicted future. Ultimately, then, you have lost your ability to be in the present moment of creation.

Often, we think by continuing the status quo ("things are good, let's keep it that way") that we are in control. But if you are focusing on the past, you will continue to just get more of what you had in the past (things were good in the past, let's keep it that way). This could be good or bad over time, but either way leaves no space for creative expansion. This becomes the status quo. When this really doesn't work for us is when we try to control life by keeping something bad in the past from happening in our present. When we focus in this manner, we are just inviting more bad happenings into the present.

If you are trying to control the future by making it turn out right, good, or better, then you are just caught up in judgment about the outcome. Inherently, there is no right or wrong, no good or bad; there is just an outcome. If you are trying to keep something bad from happening in the future, then just be present with what is right now. You can decide later if the outcome is useful or not, productive or not. If you are trying to keep something you imagine might happen in the future from happening, then stop imagining anything other than how you would love your future to be. Focus on that!

No wonder you are so damn tired all of the time. You are resisting the present, what is right in front of you right now, by trying to control the past and the future. Clues: one, the past is already gone, and you can't do anything about it now; two, the future hasn't arrived yet and is only created moment by moment in what happens in the present. But guess what? You just missed the potential unlimited creative possibilities in the present moment worrying or being obsessed with the future. Damned if we do, damned if we don't. A bit perplexing, isn't it?

One more note on control. As I learned through my journey or challenge with cancer, there is only one thing we have true control over in our lives and that is our perspective. Life will invariably lay challenges and hurdles in our path. How we choose to perceive them and then own those perceptions will make us or break us. So, no matter your challenge, exercise your power of choice with your perspective. Then, choose an empowering and inspiring perspective—and love it.

The Lower Limb, Lower Leg

The lower leg area, which includes the shin and calf, is somewhat similar to the forearm of the upper extremity. The lower leg is associated with the Action Gateway and is involved in the emotions of moving us forward and taking action in our lives. The calf, where most pain and discomfort are experienced, is about control. Imbalance in this gateway as it relates to the calf will manifest as fearing to take action, fear of the future that leads to immobilization, and inactivity. Wanting to control our movement forward or what happens in our future is a process that happens to most of us too often. When a person experiences the pain of shin splints, we often see from a Health Code perspective that they may be bumping up against an issue that is right in front of them that they are choosing to ignore. The onset of pain due to shin splints will actually slow a person down, literally, to look at whatever is in their life that needs attention. It may mean the client is stuck in growth-avoidance or excessive conservatism.

Awareness Keys

- The Action Gateway is about radiating your personal power out in the world.

- The Action Gateway gives us the actual momentum to move forward and realize our personal desires and intentions in the world.

- When the Action Gateway energy is blocked, we undermine ourself-esteem, become over-controlling. We also may feel helpless or irresponsible.

- Blocked energy in the Action Gateway could also manifest as a lack of clear direction, lack of purpose or ambition. Which may exhibit as having a lot of ideas, but finding no way to realize them.

- The stomach and spleen/pancreas are coupled meridians therefore overlap in some of their emotions.

- The stomach is about feelings of disgust. The pancreas is about self-doubt, self-criticism and not allowing the sweetness of life in.

- Adrenal glands are associated with the Action Gateway and are about exhaustion, running on empty, and being drained of life force.

- Adrenal glands are about personal expansion and formation of your identity through relating to others and the world.

- The liver can harbor the emotions of anger, resentment, irritation and frustration.

- With liver organ dysfunction we often see the emotions of anger and depression caught in a cycle, a downward spiral.

- The gallbladder is the sac that is attached to the liver. It is not a stretch of the imagination to think that unresolved anger from the liver draining into the gallbladder might turn into the hardened stones of resentment.

- The forearms are all about trying to control. The best solution to control is to realize that you can only control how you respond to whatever happens. You control your perspective. That's it.

- The lower leg, shin and calf are associated with the Action Gateway and harbor the emotions of difficulty moving forward or taking action in our lives.

- Shin splints or calf tightness will slow us down to take a look at whatever needs attention in our lives.

Chapter 10

The Pleasure Gateway

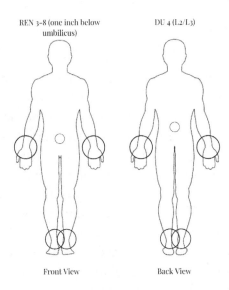

REN 3–8 (one inch below umbilicus) DU 4 (L2/L3)

Front View Back View

The Pleasure Gateway is linked to the sacral chakra, and is located just below the navel, with orange as its color. The Pleasure Gateway is associated with the emotional body, sensuality, creativity, and is directed by the principle of pleasure. It processes our emotional feelings especially involving relationships, expression of sexuality and our sensual pleasure. It balances the energy of feeling your outer and inner worlds, the ability to birth creativity and create fantasy.

Imbalances can manifest as dependency or codependency with other people or with substances that grant you easy access to pleasure. It can manifest as you being ruled by your emotions or feeling numb. A client might appear out of touch with how they feel. It might manifest as a person being overindulgent in fantasies or sexual obsessions. If blocked, it can cause a lack of sexual desire or satisfaction. A client might be feeling stuck in a particular feeling or mood and not able to get out of it.

When the Pleasure Gateway is balanced, the relationship you have with other people and with the world is centered on a harmonious and nurturing exchange of energy. An open and balanced gateway will allow you to experience intimacy and love in a fulfilling way. Creativity and a strong intuition are the benefits of a balanced gateway

Large Intestine

As I said in the Love Gateway discussion, the large intestine and lung are coupled meridians and thus linked through the acupuncture system so they share some similar emotions. However, for the Pleasure Gateway, which is associated with the large intestine, it also has its own unique emotions. The large intestine is most commonly associated with being dogmatically positioned, defensive, and compelled to neatness. Now you are probably thinking what the heck does this mean? Dogmatically positioned is about having or taking a position and not being willing to let it go. This most commonly arises when you are sure you are right and someone else's perspective is wrong. Sometimes we get in that position when we know the right thing to do is give up a stance, position, or rightness, yet we just don't or won't. That is dogmatically positioned.

Another common emotion is called compelled to neatness. On one hand, this might actually be associated with a cleanliness fetish. However, most of the time it is linked with a situation where things have gotten emotionally or situationally messy. We have a deep desire to clean things, to get things straight, and get ourselves back into integrity. Imbalances in the large intestine can manifest as being plagued by feelings of exasperation, doubt, loneliness or being left out. When these emotions play out in our life we may feel a strong inclination to throw the baby out with the bath water. This area is often associated with the "Cinderella" pattern of being used and abused, rushed, and over-controlled.

Spleen

The Pleasure Gateway is also associated with the spleen, which is our biggest lymphatic organ and is often associated with feelings of low self-esteem. The most prevalent additional emotions are lack of control over events, disgust, and hopelessness. These emotions may coincide with excessive worry and being obsessed with things. They may actually be emotions felt by a person who feels unsafe and insecure in the world. If you are showing signs of lymphatic sluggishness, such as a cold, swelling in the extremities or maybe flu-like symptoms but not actually having the flu, look to the emotions of the spleen. You might want to investigate where in your life you are feeling out of control, feeling hopeless about a situation, or where your self-esteem has recently taken a dive or a beating.

In my case, spleen emotions exhibited in conjunction with my diagnosis of lymphoma. I realized that I had created an environment for lymphoma to be expressed in my body on an emotional level as well as a physical level. The emotions I discovered were most likely because I had gotten to a place in my life where I needed, wanted, and desired to change my work. I felt that planning to change the way I approached my work was a path that would allow me to express myself in the world in a more profound way. However, my sense of low self-esteem and my feelings of lack of control over events (like my practice was running me, I was not running my practice) were taking their toll on my health. These emotions then created feelings of self-disgust and a sense of powerlessness, even hopelessness, to change things. I could not facilitate the Action Gateway to actually move forward. It was the perfect storm of emotional and mental stress to set me up for an interesting journey for which I wasn't quite prepared.

I knew I was doing it, but was not prepared for my body to give me the intensity of lymphoma as the wakeup call. I'm grateful that it happened, as weird as that may sound. My cancer experience gave me the opportunity to really look at my life and see where I needed to get back to a state of being empowered. It allowed me to find my way back to being inspired to express my gifts, talents, and abilities. What followed was some massive action. Lesson learned. I don't intend to put action off again when it comes to moving my purpose and passion forward.

Kidney, Bladder

The kidneys and bladder move fluids in the body. The kidneys are responsible for filtering the blood and cellular fluids of unwanted or toxic materials. The bladder then eliminates them from the body. If you are experiencing fear, then you are engaging the kidney meridian. Although fear is most often stored emotionally in the kidney, the emotional energy of dread, bad memory, and contemplation about some action or opportunity is also stored there. If you are experiencing fear about some upcoming event, then you might end up in the washroom urinating more often than usual. You may develop pain or discomfort in the lower thoracic to lower back area as this area of the spine or back is neurologically associated with referred stress on the kidney.

However, the kidney is also classically known for the emotion called paralyzed will. Paralyzed will is that state or emotion in which you would like to make something different, but you feel like you can't make it different, or don't know what to do to make it different. In a way, it is like being stuck. For instance, maybe you would like to make your relationship with your sister different or better, but you just can't figure out what to do to make it better.

The bladder, from a Health Code standpoint, is about being pissed off. To be more respectful, we will say it is about being miffed. Bladder is also associated with being timid or holding back in some action or opportunity. If you find yourself feeling wishy-washy about something, being unable to make a choice about it, then you may be storing this in the bladder tissue or stressing the energy of the bladder meridian. However, if you are experiencing a bladder infection, yeast infection, or potentially bladder cancer, you might want to sift through your past and find all the people that are part of your "miffed" list—especially those people on the list that you haven't let go of or forgiven yet. Clear that stuff out and get on with forgiving and relieving that bladder stress. Based on my years of working with clients, you can trust me on this one. I've seen it happen so many times.

A prime example is something my father experienced, about 30 years ago. I regret to say that my dad passed away a few months before his 101-year birthday, during the editing of this book. However, back then, my father was the sole heir to my grandmother's estate. It is a long story, but the short version is that my grandmother was in nursing care in Missouri. My dad had set up her estate to take complete care of her bills and her care in the nursing home. While my dad was busy taking care of her and traveling back and forth from his job in Texas, the grandchildren of my step- grandfather had arranged for the money in the estate and the family farms and equipment to be liquidated.

Upon my grandmother's passing, my dad was presented with a bill from the nursing home for care for the last year of her life. They told him that none of the bills had been paid over the year, that the estate had no money in it, and the farms and equipment had been transferred to my step-grandfather's children. They had crafted a way to empty the bank accounts and take over all of the leftover assets of the farms. My father is one of the kindest, most trustworthy, and reasonable men I've ever known in my life. This betrayal, and underhanded theft of my grandmother's properties, money, and assets, devastated him. I have never seen him so pissed off. He could have possibly gone after them, but was told it would take money and lots of time to prove the indiscretions. We didn't have either the money to fight or the time to invest.

Dad paid the bills and didn't take action on them, as painful as it was. Six months later he developed bladder cancer. Doctors made heroic experimental surgery on him back then, which saved his life. He was grateful, and I know as hard as it was for him, he forgave the other parties who stole from our family. That is the integrity of my father. But for our purposes here, I can state that there is no doubt in my mind that this emotional shock and internal conflict was a direct contribution to my father's bladder cancer. It's too much of a coincidence to ignore that one. This is when I first started putting these correlations of the body-mind and emotions together in my mind. I dedicate my searching and seeking, and this book, to my father and my beloved brothers

David and Chuck. My brother David left us as well, 24 hours before my father. He was a brilliant mentor and coach to me throughout my life. My father and brother were not only great men in my life but were awesome mentors and teachers for me.

The Uterus

The sex organs represent creativity in the Health Code model. Think about it. It just makes sense. Where does the creation of our offspring happen? In ancient healing methods I have studied, the sex organs are always associated with the second chakra center, which with the associated nerve plexuses and acupoints is the Pleasure Gateway. In this model, the pleasure gateway, the second chakra is considered our creative center where ideas, concepts, and creative solutions are born mentally, emotionally, and sexually. If you are suffering from low energy, dysfunction, or disease of these organs, look to balancing this gateway. You would want to strongly consider where in your life you have lost your creativity and where your creative energy is being wasted or eaten up in the process of living your life.

The emotions most associated with the sex organs being blocked are nonthinking, non-emotive, depleted, and suppressed. Non-thinking and non-emotive are expressed in what I call the "living flat-liners". In other words, "cardboard" people, those with very low affect. I'm sure you have experienced these people walking around out in the world, or worse yet, maybe someone who is currently living in your household. They are blasé, somewhat expressionless, taking a long time to respond to a simple question. Most of us refer to it as "burnt out" or "checked out." You will also know them by their lack of emotion. They don't get excited and they don't necessarily exhibit sadness or depression but appear to just be apathetic.

Emotionless as they seem, it is simply that they can't process any more energy because they are in complete exhaustion mentally, emotionally, and physically. These people often have been in a situation with another person who has been keeping them down. This has created an energy pattern of suppressing the expression of their natural gifts, talents, abilities, and their personality. Their true self has been so suppressed they have literally lost themselves. Suppression of the true self is sometimes the lowest place to be. In the patriarchal society in which we live, the uterus—including the feminine and creative—is greatly feared and devalued. Allowing your energy to resonate with this fear and devaluation of the feminine eliminates choices, options, and opportunities. When we lose our creative power we may develop feelings of sluggishness or poor memory, also emotions of the sex organs. In an effort to create energy balance, the body-mind will try to reestablish itself through the dream state. Vivid dreaming, another emotion of the sex organs, is a strong attempt of the soul to resolve this suppression cycle, to find a way back to being alive, and to return to a strong spiritual connection.

The Prostate

The prostate is an expression of the Pleasure Gateway and so is all about sensuality, relationships, expression of sexuality, sensual pleasure, birthing creativity, and creating fantasy. When men get stuck (energetically blocked) in these areas, which is often for men, then they are halting these expressions in their lives. They may be doing this in many different ways. They are often plagued by emotional tenseness or even sexual impotence due to emotional conflict. It can manifest as imbalanced when feeling that being male is a shameful thing or that they just don't cut it as a man. The emotions of the Pleasure Gateway are very charged and highly sensitive topics in our patriarchal culture. This could lead to feelings of pressure to perform sexually or concerns in addition to guilt over past carelessness. Usually, men are not good at talking about this with their partners and they often experience these things in the privacy of their minds, in secret. This is where the energy gets blocked and may create everything from benign hypertrophy (swelling of the prostate) to inflammation of the prostate (prostatitis) to cancer. All of these are signs of blocked energy not moving appropriately through the organ, meridian, and the gateway.

Low Back: Lumbar Spine

Moving right along, let's tackle the lower back area or lumbar region of the spine. This part of the spine is associated with supporting the frame of the body and maintaining the center of gravity that keeps us in balance. From an emotional standpoint, this area has to do with a person's relationship to what I call the four F's: fear, foundation (values and principles), finances, and family.

Foundational issues can be very widespread indeed. They are most often associated with whether you are, or are not, feeling supported in your life. People tend to feel various types of support. There is financial support, emotional support, or spiritual support. There is also the concept of feeling support from others or feeling like we support ourselves. All of these are dependent on how well you maintain your emotional, spiritual, and mental center of balance.

Left low back pain, strain, or discomfort is associated with emotional trauma from the past. Usually this trauma involves your family of origin and how you were supported as a child. It may be something that continues to be an issue for you with your family of origin. It may be triggered by others in your life now and whether you feel supported or not.

Are you staying with my line of thinking so far? Well, then it might be interesting to you that pain, strain, or discomfort on the right side of the lower back area is associated with the four F's in the present or future. People can experience this lack of support in the present moment, or when they are anticipating lack of support in the future. For instance, Beth came to the office for her appointment experiencing tension and anxiety. We discovered that this tension in her low back was associated with her belief that she wouldn't be able to maintain herself financially in the future. This is a common theme for many people. A large percentage of the population lives on the financial edge. Statistics suggest that most people are 30 – 90 days from bankruptcy. This may be one of the most prevalent stresses we subtly have in our everyday environment.

If we are exposed to a circumstance that threatens our belief about our financial stability, it can drive our fear of the future instantly. Beth's feeling of not being able to maintain financial independence drove her deep into emotional paralysis and physical pain. Beth is not alone in this body-mind conundrum. It is probably no coincidence that low back pain is the number one cause of pain and lost work time in our culture, at 80 million cases per year. So we know that fear is prevalent in our cultural experience, and much of the media is thriving on our fear. Foundation being about our principles and values is also always present in our day-to-day decisions. Where and how many times do you have to stand strong or compromise some of your principles and values? Family is ever present in our minds and emotions, even if we have distanced ourselves from the physical contact of our families. They live within our emotional experiences. Finances we have already talked about. Is it now more evident why low back pain is the number one place to emotionally collide with our physical body?

Often, low back pain is accompanied by sciatic pain, which is nerve pain that runs down the back of the leg. Nerve pain as a general rule is a Health Code about irritated or broken-down communication lines. If you are feeling unsupported, either emotionally or financially, this can create low back pain. If, in addition, you feel that you can't communicate adequately about this fear with whoever is involved, or they get irritated with you when you attempt to talk about it, then you may experience sciatic nerve pain down the leg as well. Really beginning to get the picture now? Let's continue.

The Ankles

The ankle and foot area, from a Health Code perspective, are associated with the ability or inability to move forward. In the Hindu system, there are specific chakras associated with the legs as I mentioned previously. The Rasatala chakra is located in the ankles and is aligned with the emotions of selfishness and charity. So, again we see that if you are paying attention to your own selfishness and not the feelings of others in a situation, where you are walking all over them or trying to control them, you could be having ankle pain or strain that is present in response to your chakra energy being out of balance.

The ankles are associated with the Pleasure Gateway and sacral chakra as well. So all of the concepts of being flexible and moving forward can be co-mingled with the emotions of the Pleasure Gateway. For example, the Pleasure Gateway is about creativity, relationships and having access to pleasure. If we are having pain or inflexibility in our ankle, then we are likely getting stuck in our codependence in a relationship that is making us feel numb or out of touch with how we feel. This may appear as a lack of sexual desire or satisfaction. It may also manifest as being too accommodating, cooperative, understanding, and respectful of the opinions and beliefs of others. If you are having ankle problems, you may be having difficulty advancing towards your own goals. It may be that you have illusions of self-inflation concerning your goals and objectives.

The Wrist

The wrist is associated with the Pleasure Gateway, which again is about sensuality, creativity, and directed by the principles of pleasure. It can manifest as being ruled by our emotions and feeling out of touch with how you feel. It makes sense that carpal tunnel syndrome, which is a numbness in the hands that originates in the wrist, is the manifestation of an unbalanced gateway. This unbalanced gateway is exhibiting being out of touch with your feelings, numbing out, and feeling stuck. I will add here that the expression of numbness in the arm, forearm, and hands is a combination of overlapping emotions. This blocked energy could extend from the neck, shoulder, upper arm, elbow, forearm, wrist, or hand. So to look at it from a view of all of these areas might be highly significant.

If pain or blockage is involving a number of Chakra centers and emotional gateways throughout the arm, then you will need to look at all segments. Then determine the story that is being told by your body and mind through your unbalanced emotions. Wrist problems can manifest as a person having difficulty articulating and carrying out their intentions. They may also be concerned about their ability to move through life with ease and skill. This may show up as them being rather ungraceful and uptight in their execution of things. Often I see that clients are holding themselves back from their full expression. Often there is something they should be doing or that they want to be doing, but they aren't doing it. Last, but by far not least, the emotions that are more prevalent when this area is blocked range from being highly sensitive to criticism, craving recognition, demanding appreciation, and wanting a response from the world around them.

Awareness Keys

- The Pleasure Gateway imbalance can manifest as being out of touch with your feelings. An overactive gateway may show up in creating unhealthy relationships or unhealthy addictions.

- The Pleasure Gateway is associated with the emotional body, sensuality, and creativity.

- Physical symptoms of an overactive Pleasure Gateway can be gynecological problems, lower back pain, kidney problems, or urinary issues.

- The large intestine is associated with being dogmatically positioned, defensive or compelled to neatness. You may also have stuck energy in the large intestine when you are feeling exasperated, lonely or left out.

- The spleen harbors the emotions of lack of control over events, feelings of hopelessness and disgust.

- Kidneys are emotionally associated with fear and paralyzed will. Paralyzed will being, "wanting something to be different but can figure out what to do, or how to make it different."

- Bladder is emotionally about being "pissed off" or "miffed."

- The uterus is where our mental, emotional and sexual creative energy arises.

- The uterus is also where feelings of non-emotive, depleted, and suppression are carried.

- When the true expressions of our gifts, talents and abilities have been suppressed so long we literally lose ourselves.

- When the energy of the prostate is blocked, men are plagued by emotional tenseness. Often this shows up as sexual impotence.

- This blocked Pleasure Gateway energy can occur with the emotions of shame, pressure to perform sexually or with guilt.

- Low back pain is all about the four F's: fear, foundation (your values and principles), finances and family.

- The ankles are about your ability or inability to move forward in life.

- The ankle is also the area of where there is a conflict of emotions between selfishness and charity

- The wrists are associated with sensitivity to criticism, craving recognition, feeling out of touch with how you feel, and numbed out.

Chapter 11

The Foundation Gateway

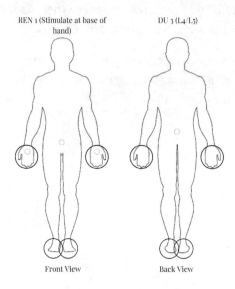

REN 1 (Stimulate at base of hand)

DU 3 (L4/L5)

Front View   Back View

The Foundation Gateway, which is harmonious with the root chakra, is located in the lower pelvis and at the base of spine. Its color is red. It is about safety and grounding (safe versus vulnerable or being at risk). It lays the foundation for expansion in your life. It supports us in growing and feeling safe into exploring all the aspects of life. I relate it to the 4 F's: fear, foundation, family, and finances.

The characteristics for the Foundation Gateway are associated with security, safety, survival, and basic needs (food, sleep, shelter, self-preservation). It is associated with physicality, physical identity, grounding, support, and the foundation for living our lives. This gateway is where we ground ourselves into the earth and anchor our energy into the manifest world. For a person who is unbalanced in this gateway it might be hard for them to feel safe in the world. They may feel like everything looks or feels like a potential risk. When this gateway is blocked, a person's behaviors will be ruled mainly by fear. If there is an excess of energy in this gateway their behavior might show up as greed or paranoia. This can often manifest as issues like over-controlling food intake and obsessiveness around their diet.

Balancing this gateway is best done with earth type activities. For example, hiking, gardening, connecting with nature or even cooking healthy meals. As I mentioned above, this is the foundation part of the 4F's. It is associated with our personal values and principles. This gateway helps us stay balanced in honoring and living from these values and principles. It is also where we get blocked when we find ourselves compromising or blatantly disregarding our values and principles.

Ovaries, Testicles

The sex organs, ovaries, and testicles again represent creativity in the Health Code model. While researching and aligning these principles, I found the ancient healing methods associate the ovaries and testicles with the Foundation Gateway; the first chakra center. In this system of energy, the Foundation Gateway is considered our safety and security center. It is where the energy of ideas, concepts, and creative solutions are allowed to thrive in a foundation of safety. If you are suffering from low energy, dysfunction, or disease of these organs, then you would want to strongly consider where in your life you have lost your feelings of safety, support, and how you are feeling a diminished sense of physicality.

The emotions most associated with the sex organs when they are imbalanced are non-thinking, non-emotive, depleted, and suppressed. Non-thinking and non-emotive are manifested often times because we don't feel safe expressing our true self. We may feel impotent to apply our ideas, thoughts, and take actions that challenge the status quo. Like the sexual organs of the Pleasure Gateway/second chakra, this need for safety and self-preservation may manifest as a person being blasé, somewhat expressionless, or even taking a long time to respond to a simple question.

Sacrum, Coccyx, and Pelvis

The sacrum and coccyx at the bottom tip of the spine, our tail-bone and pelvis all are associated with the Foundation Gateway, the first chakra. It is associated with the emotion of fear. What happens when a dog has just been scared or scolded? He tucks his tail and runs. It's common in our culture to be scolded or to be frightened and to want to tuck our tails and run. Unfortunately, tucking your tail and running is generally not considered socially acceptable behavior. Instead, we stand there and take the scolding, acting macho and unafraid. Later, you may end up with low back pain or a pain in your butt. The phrase "so-and-so is a pain in the ass!" takes on a whole new meaning in this emotional setting. This demonstrates why the sacrum and coccyx are most often associated with unexpressed and unresolved stress from a fearful situation or reprimand.

In addition, the sacrum and coccyx are very much associated with the cranial sacral pump mechanism. This rhythmic pulsation between the cranium (the bones of the skull) and the sacrum is responsible for the flow of cerebral spinal fluid up and down the spinal canal. This fluid bathes the central nervous system with oxygen, nutrients, and glucose. The sacral area is also associated with the foundational energy center of the body and supports the whole system of the central nervous system. When the sacrum is blocked, in dysfunction, or pain, it may be an indication of an inability to balance head, heart, and pelvis.

Pain in this region can include long-held beliefs, traumas, or incongruences. Emotionally, it is a representation of foundational issues (values, principles, beliefs, and life scripts) as well as generational or ancestral energy patterns. These ancestral energies are handed down genetically and become part of our habitual behavior patterns. The problem is these old energy patterns may not serve you at this time in your life. An example may be that you grew up in a family where women were considered less powerful, that they should stay quiet on matters of life, principle, and power. However, you may now be a CEO of a major corporation or a single parent raising a family. These jobs in my estimation are not dissimilar. Now that you are being called upon to step into your power, to generate change, or even survive, this incongruent energy from past beliefs is stuck in pain or dysfunction in the sacral area. This is where you might want to bring your attention and your awareness to the thought that it may be time to shift this belief. It may be time to change this behavior and be open to healing some deeper wounds.

A clinical example of this comes to mind with a female client of mine, Ari, who was a powerful corporate upper management leader. She was having consistent episodes of sacral pain and pelvic pain as well as frequent headaches. In our work together, we discovered that she was very discontented with her work. She felt out of her natural flow and rhythm doing the work in which she had been engaged for the last 15 years. Though highly skilled, she felt like her heart was urging her in a different direction.

Growing up in a disempowering family relationship of disrespect, shame, and violence, she vowed to be powerful in her life She thought that developing a powerful persona (a personality of prestige and strength) was the solution to that life script. For years she worked to become this upper management corporate leader. However, she discovered that her heart's desire was to be powerful within herself not in her outer world. She soon quit her corporate job and went to massage school. Through our work she began to heal her past programming. With this work she found her personal power by learning to honor the natural flow in her life. She healed her headaches and her sacral and pelvic pain disappeared. She identified and worked her way emotionally back to her authentic foundation and power by discovering her value at a soul level. Today, she is an international teacher/trainer in cranial/ sacral therapy. She is a leader in helping others find their own flow and the power of their own authenticity.

The Hand and Fingers

Hands are about holding on to things or holding too tightly to things. Hands metaphorically represent our ability to grasp or get a handle on a specific situation or circumstance. We have all experienced this before and have probably heard ourselves say, "I just can't get a handle on this problem." Sometimes we have such a grip on a situation or circumstance that we are literally holding it with a "death grip". We sometimes do this in relationships that seem to be slipping away. The problem is that in the case of a relationship, it makes the situation worse and drives the other person further from us. Hands and fingers also represent handling the details of life. Often the details of life (daily grind) interfere with us finding who we are in life. When imbalanced, it can exhibit as difficulty in direction setting and integrating personal values. Often there are also concerns about social standing, power, and prestige.

As I stated above, fingers are associated with the details of life and we find ourselves injuring our fingers often. The possible insight here is stumbling or bumping up against the minutia of the day-to-day can be painful and problematic. The circumstances of life often get in our way when we are trying to push forward through achievement or accomplishment. Often, we find ourselves grasping for more money, time, love, or material things with reckless abandon.

A common complaint in my office is a condition most people have heard of: carpal tunnel syndrome. It has become more common over the last decade. I find it interesting that many of my patients feel the deep need to grasp for more. Our current culture operates under the belief that there is never enough, more is better, and that is just the way it is. This way of thinking creates a block to our deeper understanding of the way the Universe works. The result of this way of thinking gets played out in our body in the form of tension in our forearms wrist and hands that is subconscious. I see this in patients when they are on my table, supposedly relaxing, yet they have their fist clenched tight. Often just lightly tapping their fist and whispering in to them, "there is enough, you are enough, less is more and remember we live in an abundant universe, just let go and open your hand and let the energy of abundance into your life," brings deep relaxation to their entire body. Often, they spontaneously break out into laughter and say, "Thanks for the reminder."

As you move through your day, notice the tension in your hands and fingers and just stop, laugh and let go of that belief that there is not enough. Let go of that thought that you are not enough. Then smile, and maybe even laugh at yourself.

The Feet

The foot is somewhat more classically broken down into fragments. If you have pain on the top of the foot, it would be appropriate with what you now know to inquire about where you feel you are being "stepped on or walked on." If perhaps you are suffering from pain on the bottom of the foot, plantar fasciitis, or heel spurs, you might want to inquire as to whom you are stepping on or walking all over. You may need to think about whose feelings you are trampling on or even what is the irritation that is under-foot for you. In other words, what are you overlooking when it comes to other's feelings?

Again, in the Hindu system of chakras, the *patala,* located in the soles of the feet, are aligned with malice and hatred as well as forgiveness. Is there a situation that is an irritation that you are purposefully ignoring, and you are walking around the issue? Possibly it is one of those situations in which you feel you are "walking on eggshells" or feel you are "walking on thin ice." Catch my drift? In the Hindu chakras, mahatala is located more centrally in the feet near the arches and are aligned with the sense of entitlement as well as lack of a conscience, but also with expansiveness.

Toes in this conversation are about the details of life as are the fingers. The toes are associated with supporting your forward movement in life. Toes may be about not paying attention to the details of life as they pertain to your future, especially your future success in whatever endeavor lies before you. The feet are part of the Foundation Gateway, so will always be associated with laying down the foundation for expansion in your life. The feet because of the Foundation Gateway are about security, safety, survival, and grounding. This, of course, if imbalanced will manifest as feelings of insecurity, excessive negativity, cynicism, greed, or fear.

Awareness Keys

- The Foundation Gateway is about safety and grounding. It supports us in growing and feeling safe when exploring all aspects of life.

- The Foundation Gateway is about the values and principles we choose in life. Imbalance can happen when we don't honor our principles and values.

- The ovaries and testicles are where we harbor energy for ideas, concepts, and creative solutions to thrive.

- When the energy of the ovaries and testicles is blocked, this often leads to a suppression of our true self. It can limit our choices, personal power, and leave us with a loss of identity.

- The sacrum and pelvis can harbor fear but are also the seat of values, principles, beliefs, and life scripts.

- The sacrum and pelvis may contain the ancestral energy patterns that have been handed down to us over generations. These generational behaviors may not serve us so well at this point in our life.

- Hands are emotionally about holding on to things or holding too tightly to things.

- Fingers are associated with the details of life. The daily grind of duties and responsibilities.

- Remember to notice the tension in your hands and fingers during the day. Take a breath and let go of the tension. Remind yourself that it is an abundant Universe, there is enough, and you are enough.

- The foot is emotionally segmented out. The top of the foot associated with the feelings of being "stepped on" or "walked on".

- The bottom of the foot is associated with who you may be stepping on or whose feelings you are trampling on. It is the balance of emotional energy between malice and hatred versus forgiveness.

- The toes are again like the fingers, relating to the details of life.

- Toes, being part of the Foundation Gateway, are about the foundation for expansion in your life. They are about security, safety, survival, and grounding.

Chapter 12
Putting it All Together

The Universe works on one principle that seems to elude most of us: flow. The Universe likes things to stay in constant motion, to come and go like the water in a flowing river. Danielle LaPorte states it best, "going with the flow is responding to cues from the Universe. When you go with the flow, you're surfing life force. It's about wakeful trust and total collaboration with what's showing up for you." Life is this way. Life is a constant flow of experiences, opportunities, emotions, thoughts, transitions, and chances. Being in the flow means being aware that the river of life is flowing to us at every moment. Existing in a state of being is accepting whatever comes and putting it to good use. Going with the flow means allowing whatever comes to move through you freely.

Therefore, gripping tightly or trying to "trap" the flow of energy is counterproductive as far as the Universe is concerned. A problem presented in this moment then released in the next moment may present the answer to the problem in the next moment. If you are holding on so tightly to the problem from the last moment that you can't grasp the solution or answer in the next moment, then you are only left with the original problem. Let go.

You have heard this throughout this book, just let go and experience the next moment. Many of you are probably saying, "I just can't get a grasp on some of the messages in this book." You will if you allow yourself to quit trying so hard. Relax your forearms, hands, fingers, and release your grasp. My objective is to help you understand how all this goes together. If we link a number of the connected parts of the body with affiliated symptom syndromes, we can see how things in the body can create a story. Through the Health Code, we have learned that the neck is about "sticking your neck out," or about being flexible in life (or about not being flexible). We know the neck is about being able to (or not) turn and look behind at your past trauma (or look ahead at your future fears). The neck relates well to the shoulder. As the old song goes, "the neck bone is connected to the shoulder bone, and the shoulder bone is connected to the arm bone . . ."

Continuing the example, many people suffer from neck pain, with pain radiating into the shoulder and down the arm to the elbow or hand. Now, you know through the Health Code that there is a whole unique story behind this malady. Here is just one possibility in the midst of an infinite number of possibilities. The person in question, let's say, is experiencing pain on the left side of their body. Let's call her Rose, and she is struggling with an issue from her past that is currently being agitated in her relationship with the man she loves. Rose feels she has lost some flexibility around being who she wants to be, or she thinks she can be. She is experiencing emotional stress because she is afraid of not being accepted for who she is by the man she loves. In other words, she feels like she is not using her natural gifts and talents to her best ability but fears not being accepted if she does.

Rose then ends up carrying a chip on her shoulder about it toward her mate. She has a story that she can't be the best version of herself because she has too many responsibilities as a wife, mother, or girlfriend. Rose feels that if she were really herself that it would compromise her relationship or worse, maybe even bring her relationship to an end. Living in this suppression of self has affected her ability to be carefree and spontaneous. This has ultimately taken the fun out of life and so she begins to lose spontaneity, flexibility, and the humor in life. When we lose the humor, we tend to become more cynical, irritated, and much less tolerant of ourselves in addition to others. We lose our ability to love ourselves and others unconditionally, which creates more inflexibility. This erodes our communication lines with others as well as with our spiritual connection. The end result is Rose has stopped being (or expressing) the best version of herself.

Here is another possibility from a strictly physical manifestation. Someone is experiencing neck pain or stiffness, leading to shoulder pain and stiffness. If unattended long enough without being addressed, it will lead to upper arm pain radiating to the elbow or hand. The neck and shoulder areas harbor the emotions of expression as well as the conflicts between the heart and head. The elbow area, remember, is associated in the Health Code with being able to bend or be flexible. It is the area mainly associated with unconditional love issues toward others or self. Then finally with the pain comes numbness and tingling in the arm, wrist and hand, metaphorically signifying broken or irritated communication lines.

If you wanted to follow the outcome of this "rest of the story" example, it might go like this: Applying the Health Code to this patient, let's call him Jon, tells us that he has a conflict between something he feels in his heart he wants to say or do and what his mind is telling him not to. This may be his cultural programming or how he was trained to behave in his family environment. This conflict is at least causing him to suppress his true feelings, which might make him feel vulnerable. Since he is not expressing his true feelings or true self, his shoulder pain and stiffness symptoms are trying to get his attention. As mentioned above, his elbow involvement in this symptom story is an indicator that he is not unconditionally loving himself and therefore allowing himself to be his true self out in the world. With this energy pattern building up in his system, he is wanting to over-control or to be in control of others or if nothing else, at least control his own feelings and vulnerabilities. This is the emotional manifestation of the forearm. If left unattended, this manifestation can lead to pain, numbness, or dysfunction in the hand and fingers. Hands, according to the Health Code, are about getting a grasp on things, getting a handle on them. Sometimes it can be about holding on too tightly to the control you are trying to exert over someone or a situation. Now perhaps you can see this progression of events in someone you know, maybe even how you process things yourself. This is just an example and may not be how your own body processes this emotion. However, if you were experiencing these symptoms and you knew this way of looking at it, it might be just the insight or story that you need to push through the symptoms (meaning process and push out that stagnant festering energy block). It might be the exact strategy for changing this issue. It might even change the way you process a similar problem in the future. Beginning to make sense at this point? I hope so.

Another example of putting all of this together into an insightful story might go something like this. Sue comes to the office complaining of knee pain and pain in the calf. This could be that she decided to take up running again after not running for oh, let's say, three years. If Sue had not done anything, she could remember to injure that area directly, then she might want to consider her emotional Health Code. We could explore how emotionally her need to control a relationship in her life has caused her to become unyielding or unbending. In the Health Code remember the knee is associated with inflexibility and unconditional love issues. Sue might examine where in one of her relationships there has been a lack of unconditional love for another person (with unconditional meaning the ability to just accept the other person for how they are, without feeling the need to change them in some way).

Sue could evaluate if she is living out this emotional conflict by staying in the relationship. Possibly she has forced the end of the relationship and caused them to painfully move on in their life. Both of these story lines could be represented in her symptom picture as pain or tightness in the calf. Staying in the relationship showing up as tension or pain or moving on, moving forward being the calf pain. Another possibility is maybe her inability to unconditionally love herself has caused her to not have permission in her mind to move forward. Her lack of unconditional love for herself might limit her choices or ability to step into a new job, relationship, or opportunity. As you can see when you begin to play with these insights, you can find a multitude of ways in which they may relate to what is going on for you. So, you can either stay both stuck in your stuff and feel totally powerless against your circumstances or you can begin to apply some of the techniques outlined in this book.

You always have the choice, as Sue did, to eliminate your limiting beliefs, reset your perspective, and follow your vision for yourself. Choose to empower yourself: no one else is going to do it for you. This happened in Sue's case, she left the relationship, chose a new career path and ended up as my wife. We have been happily married for 30 years at the writing of this book. As Sue's mom would so often say, "How about them apples?" One additional note that you may have already figured out from our previous discussion is that often in these cases the insight can have a second element. If there is nerve pain, numbness, or tingling in the lower leg area it is associated with irritated or broken-down communications. These lines of communication can be between parts of yourself, from other gateways and chakras, or between people in your life. When there is conflict like this in relationships, often communication is what ultimately breaks down.

Here is yet another example. Eric was a young hard-working man in his early 40s when I first met him. He complained of low back and right leg sciatica. His x-rays were nearly perfect, meaning no signs of disc disease or early arthritic change. He had no history of trauma or strain injury to his low back. When we explored the muscle tension and pain on palpation and on soft tissue treatment, he had all the implications of muscle splinting or guarding.

When I introduced him to the possible emotional component of his pain, he was not impressed at first. However, with further exploration, we discovered that Eric's girlfriend was putting financial demands on Eric's budget that were a bit beyond his reach. In order to keep his status with his girlfriend, he continued to go against his inner urgings to tell her the truth about the financial strain and hardship. I explained to Eric that low back is associated with the 4F's. I told him that emotionally nerve pain (sciatica in his case) is a symptom of broken communication lines between he and his girlfriend. I also added that maybe there was a part of him that was not communicating with another aspect of his personality. I continued by saying, a part of you, your financially responsible self is in conflict with the part of you that has been taught to be a good provider at all cost. He decided to work with me, and we cleared the emotions. We cleared the emotions and beliefs he was carrying about not "being enough" and also the belief that he doesn't have value unless he is giving and providing for those around him. We also found it rewarding to clear his emotion of pride around having a beautiful young girlfriend on his arm.

He finally broke down and had the much-needed conversation with his girlfriend. The end of the story is she left him. However, what he realized was how shallow her perception was of life and of him. He actually was glad to be done with this relationship and went on to fall in love and marry a woman with a healthy respect for life and great financial values. He continues to be free of back pain and sciatica. Once he had that tough conversation where he spoke his truth and honored his values, the trapped sour energy was released, and he could move forward.

Interpretations

Hopefully, you can begin to see how the symptoms you or your patients experience in your body have significance and give more insight into the deeper meaning of life. Your body is trying to tell you something. You can choose to ignore it or you can use this information as guidance. If your body is having symptoms, then your body is feeling stress and imbalance. You can choose to listen to the gentle whispers that your body offers you and make changes in your life. If you do this and take action to change your behaviors, you will bring your life and your body back into balance. If you bring your life back to balance when you hear a whisper, then your body won't have to resort to shouting in order to get your attention. Shouting in a metaphorical sense means making symptoms stronger, longer, or more intense. My experience with cancer was a perfect example of me not listening to the whispers of my inner voice telling me to make a change in my life. It took the shouting of a critical situation for me to pay attention (and I know better than to ignore the whispers). Just goes to show that knowing something and putting it into conscious action in one's life are not the same. I state this so that as practitioners it is important to pay attention to your own wellness. As you use this information for your healing, you will actually own these principles and it will be so much easier to share your experiences with your clients as you help them heal. By being your own best physician, you enhance your effectiveness as a healer for everyone you work with.

In an effort to give you a short review and a quick reference for the areas of the body, gateways, chakra systems, and how they are associated, I am including this guide. There are some variations in this graph from the bulk of information that was covered earlier for each region of the body to give you a broader reference to what emotional meaning each area can have associated with it. Think of this as an expansion of the information and quick reference guide to what is already contained in the earlier chapters.

Body Areas and Related Emotions Chart

Basic Emotional Body Geography

- Left: Past
- Right: Present or anticipation of future
- Front: Future
- Back: Past
- Up: Spiritual
- Down: Grounding

Examples:

Left-head pain would indicate confusion or an overwhelming feeling from a past experience, whereas right-head pain would indicate confusion or an overwhelming feeling that concerns some future decision or the anticipation of something you know is happening in the future (job or career change), life changing event (birth of a child, marriage). Pain in the front of the chest indicates not being able to express your authentic self about something that is approaching in your future.

Pain in the back of the chest or ribs indicates there is something in your past that is being suppressed by someone else or by yourself. It is an indicator that your heart center isn't allowing you to receive feelings of love into your life. You may not be willing to receive the fullness of the experience.

Up, meaning any pain above the diaphragm, is an indication of things that relate to your deeper spiritual process. Anything below the diaphragm will indicate a need for grounding or more focus on the foundation of your true self.

Body Area/Gateway/Chakra Essential Oil/Yoga Pose	Associated Emotions/ Possible Connection
HEAD: *Connection Gateway/ Crown Chakra* **EO:** *frankincense, sandalwood, saffron, lotus, jasmine, lemon, rosewood* **YOGA POSE:** *Headstand, half lotus, corpse*	Confusion, overwhelming feeling, overly rational (too much in your head), operating from cultural programming that limits the expression of your authenticity.
NECK: *Expression Gateway/ Throat Chakra* **EO:** *eucalyptus, rosemary, lime, sage, cedarwood, peppermint, cypress, chamomile* **YOGA POSE:** *shoulder stand, camel, plow, bridge*	Conflict between your head and heart, letting your rational thinking have more power than your heart's passion and purpose.
CHEST/RIBS: *Love Gateway/ Heart Chakra* **EO:** *geranium, lime, spearmint, rose essential, ylang ylang, jasmine, eucalyptus* **YOGA POSE:** *back bend, eagle*	Not taking in the fullness of life, not breathing in the spirit of who you are at your essence.
MIDBACK: *Love Gateway/ Heart Chakra* **EO:** *geranium, lime, spearmint, rose essential, ylang ylang, jasmine, eucalyptus* **YOGA POSE:** *back bend, eagle*	Anger, frustration, irritation or resentment that is holding you back from living your heart's desire.

Body Area/Gateway/Chakra Essential Oil/Yoga Pose	Associated Emotions/ Possible Connection
SHOULDERS: *Vision Gateway/3rd Eye Chakra* **EO:** *lavender, jasmine, myrrh, patchouli, basil, sandalwood, frankincense, clary sage* **YOGA POSE:** *shoulder stand, cat/cow, child*	Unexpressed emotion or an aspect of you that is not being expressed (creativity, a gift, talent or ability).
UPPER ARM: *Expression Gateway/Throat Chakra* **EO:** *eucalyptus, rosemary, lime, sage, cedarwood, peppermint, cypress, chamomile* **YOGA POSE:** *shoulder stand, camel, plow, bridge*	Taking life or a circumstance too seriously, not finding the humor in a situation or circumstance.
FOREARM: *Action Gateway/ Solar Chakra* **EO:** *cedarwood, grapefruit, sweet marjoram, black pepper* **YOGA POSE:** *sun salutation, boat, leg lifts, mountain*	Trying too much to control a situation or circumstance, gripping too tightly to something, or holding on too tightly
ELBOW: *Love Gateway/Heart Chakra* **EO:** *geranium, lime, spearmint, rose essential, ylang ylang, jasmine, eucalyptus* **YOGA POSE:** *back bend, eagle*	Not allowing unconditional love of self, or not giving unconditional love to another.

Body Area/Gateway/Chakra Essential Oil/Yoga Pose	Associated Emotions/ Possible Connection
WRIST: *Pleasure Gateway/ Sacral Chakra* **EO:** *ylang ylang, sandalwood, jasmine, bergamot, clary sage, neroli, cardamom* **YOGA POSE:** *cow face, pigeon, bound and open angle*	Control and inability to be flexible with self or others. Gripping and holding on when it would be best to just let go.
HAND: *Foundation Gateway/ Root Chakra* **EO:** *vetiver, myrrh, frankincense, grapefruit, pine, ginger, ylang ylang, rosewood, black pepper* **YOGA POSE:** *reclining bound angle, child, forward bend, head to knee*	Control and inability to be flexible with self or others. Gripping and holding on when it would be best to just let go.
FINGERS: *Foundation Gateway/Root Chakra* **EO:** *vetiver, myrrh, frankincense, grapefruit, pine, ginger, ylang ylang, rosewood, black pepper* **YOGA POSE:** *reclining bound angle, child, forward bend, head to knee*	Being too concerned with the details of life. Not allowing the natural flow and the unfolding of the natural process of things.
ABDOMEN: *Action Gateway/ Solar Chakra* **EO:** *cedarwood, grapefruit, sweet marjoram, black pepper* **YOGA POSE:** *sun salutation, boat, leg lifts, mountain*	Ignoring a gut feeling, not listening to intuition.

Body Area/Gateway/Chakra Essential Oil/Yoga Pose	Associated Emotions/ Possible Connection
LOW BACK: *Pleasure Gateway/Sacral Chakra* **EO:** *ylang ylang, sandalwood, jasmine, bergamot, clary sage, neroli, cardamom* **YOGA POSE:** *cow face, pigeon, bound and open angle*	A problem in your life with one or more of the 4 F's, Fear, Finances, Family, or Foundation (your principles and values).
PELVIS: *Foundation Gateway/Root Chakra* **EO:** *vetiver, myrrh, frankincense, grapefruit, pine, ginger, ylang ylang, rosewood, black pepper* **YOGA POSE:** *reclining bound angle, child, forward bend, head to knee*	A conflict with your creative expression, your foundational beliefs (principles and values) and your sexual nature or expression.
HIPS: *Vision Gateway/3rd Eye Chakra* **EO:** *lavender, jasmine, myrrh, patchouli, basil, sandalwood, frankincense, clary sage* **YOGA POSE:** *shoulder stand, cat/cow, child*	Holding back in your personal expression and expressing who you are at your core.
UPPER LEG/THIGH: *Expression Gateway/Throat Chakra* **EO:** *eucalyptus, rosemary, lime, sage, cedarwood, peppermint, cypress, chamomile* **YOGA POSE:** *shoulder stand, camel, plow, bridge*	Difficulty moving forward or holding on too much to your limitation from the past. Feeling stuck by some mistake or situation that you regret from your past that doesn't let you move forward.

Body Area/Gateway/Chakra Essential Oil/Yoga Pose	Associated Emotions/ Possible Connection
KNEE: *Love Gateway/Heart Chakra* **EO:** *geranium, lime, spearmint, rose essential, ylang ylang, jasmine, eucalyptus* **YOGA POSE:** *back bend, eagle*	Being too flexible (bending over backward) or not being flexible enough in a situation that requires you to love unconditionally (either yourself or someone else).
LOWER LEG/CALF: *Action Gateway/Solar Chakra* **EO:** *cedarwood, grapefruit, sweet marjoram, black pepper* **YOGA POSE:** *sun salutation, boat, leg lifts, mountain*	Not allowing yourself the safety to jump into the next stage of life, business, or a relationship based on fear.
ANKLE: *Pleasure Gateway/ Sacral Chakra* **EO:** *ylang ylang, sandalwood, jasmine, bergamot, clary sage, neroli, cardamom* **YOGA POSE:** *cow face, pigeon, bound and open angle*	Control over your foundational beliefs. A belief about yourself or the world that may not be true, however, you don't trust yourself enough to open to a new belief.
FOOT: *Foundation Gateway/ Root Chakra* **EO:** *vetiver, myrrh, frankincense, grapefruit, pine, ginger, ylang ylang, rosewood, black pepper* **YOGA POSE:** *reclining bound angle, child, forward bend, head to knee*	You are not paying attention to or you are not hearing the whispers of your soul. Your current path is out of sync with who you are and where you are going.

Body Area/Gateway/Chakra Essential Oil/Yoga Pose	Associated Emotions/ Possible Connection
TOES: *Foundation Gateway/ Root Chakra* **EO:** *vetiver, myrrh, frankincense, grapefruit, pine, ginger, ylang ylang, rosewood, black pepper* **YOGA POSE:** *reclining bound angle, child, forward bend, head to knee*	Too strictly adhering to the details of the task in front of you and not allowing yourself to clearly see and trust the unfolding of your path ahead.

The Organ Systems (The Inside Stories)

Basic Internal Organ Anatomy

Most of the internal organ systems in the body are found in the mid-line of the body and between the top of the head and lower aspect of the pelvis (called the pelvic floor). There are those organs found above the respiratory diaphragm in our head, neck, and chest and the organs below in our abdomen and pelvis. Organs discussed above the diaphragm included the lungs, heart, thyroid, pineal gland, pituitary gland, and thymus. Those below the diaphragm included the liver, gallbladder, stomach, pancreas, small intestine, large intestine, spleen, kidneys, adrenals, bladder, and sex organs (including ovaries, uterus, and testes).

When we look to the subtle systems, the bio-emotional gateways, the acupuncture system, nervous system and chakra system, we find that these systems are interrelated. These subtle energy systems often orchestrate the proper functioning of the body in a purposeful symphony. The acupuncture system breaks these organ systems into a relationship of coupled meridians. These coupled meridians work energetically with each other to maintain a powerful balance within the body. The acupuncture meridian is named for the organ it goes to or through as it travels through its course in the body. Examples are liver meridian and the liver, lung meridian and the lung, etc.

The chart included with this section categorizes the different organ systems in their coupled meridian sequences. Each organ is associated with the gateway and chakra it is linked to in the subtle energy systems. It also outlines the basic emotions associated with each organ. The most common emotions in each group are called the primary emotions, which are those emotions most commonly imbalanced and associated with that organ or meridian. However, we often find the secondary emotions, which are additional Health Code emotions that are significant and just as important when we go looking for blockages. Both sets of emotions limit our ability to move forward during a challenging time in our life. Stay open and curious as to what might fit or be playing out in your own situation or circumstance. If you have an intuitive feeling about it, you are probably right! Trust it and go with that.

Organ Systems and Emotions Chart

Organ	Primary Emotions	Secondary Emotions
STOMACH *Action Gateway* *Solar plexus chakra*	Over sympathetic	Disgust, expanded self-importance, despair, nervous, obsessive, egotistic, stifled, unreliable, inferiority
SPLEEN *Pleasure Gateway* *Sacral chakra*	Low self-esteem, useless	Lives through others, over concern, hopeless, lacking control, worried
PANCREAS *Action Gateway* *Solar plexus chakra*	Self-criticism	Distrust, rejected, rejecting, feeling unaccepted

Organ	Primary Emotions	Secondary Emotions
LUNG *Love Gateway* *Heart chakra*	Grief	Sadness, yearning, cloudy thinking, anguish
LARGE INTESTINE *Pleasure Gateway* *Sacral chakra*	Dogmatically positioned	Crying, compelled to neatness, defensive, doubt, exasperated, lonely, left out
KIDNEY *Pleasure Gateway* *Sacral chakra*	Fear	Dread, bad memory, contemplative, disloyal, betrayal, betrayed
BLADDER *Pleasure Gateway* *Sacral chakra*	Paralyzed will	Miffed, timid, inefficient, wishy-washy, "comme çi, comme ça", futile
GALLBLADDER *Action Gateway* *Solar plexus chakra*	Resentment	Galled, stubborn, emotionally repressed, depressed, indecisive
LIVER *Action Gateway* *Solar plexus chakra*	Anger	Irrational, frustrated, aggressive
HEART *Love Gateway* *Heart chakra*	Frightfully overjoyed	Uncomfortable laughing, lacking emotion, feeling antsy, inability to be with an emotion or to sit still

Organ	Primary Emotions	Secondary Emotions
SMALL INTESTINE *Action Gateway* *Solar plexus chakra*	Lost, vulnerable, unappreciated	Deserted, abandoned, absent mindedness, insecurity, profoundly deep unrequited love
THYROID *Expression Gateway* *Throat chakra* **ADRENALS** *Action Gateway* *Solar plexus chakra*	Shamed, humiliated, muddle instability Used, anxious	Irritated, paranoia, muddled thinking, emotional instability, up and down, can't figure it out
PROSTATE, UTERUS *Pleasure Gateway* *Sacral chakra* **TESTICLES, OVARIES** *Foundation Gateway* *Root chakra*	Non-thinking, non-emotive, unfulfilled Depleted, suppressed	Sluggish memory, vivid dreaming
PITUITARY *Connection Gateway* *Crown chakra*	Disappointment	Inflexible, belligerent Speechless, spiritually disconnected
PINEAL *Vision Gateway* *Third eye chakra*	Unclear vision, can't see ahead clearly	Speechless, spiritually disconnected

Organ	Primary Emotions	Secondary Emotions
THYMUS *Love Gateway* *Heart chakra*	Resignation, resigning yourself	Troubled, overwhelmed, attacked, attacking

This next section is a compilation of therapies you can apply directly to the bio-emotional gateway centers. I have brought together self-care remedies that I have found effective for balancing the gateways and neutralizing the emotional energy associated with each of the seven gateways. You are free to share these with your patients, as you see appropriate as a healer. You can help them learn to identify through their intuition what the emotion is that they are stuck in or that is blocking the flow of energy in their life. You as a healer can explore and experiment with this as well on your own challenges.

Healers that use muscle testing methods:

If you are a practitioner that uses muscle-testing techniques in your work, then you can actually just test each gateway center to find the imbalanced gateway. Once you know that then you can use the charts from earlier in this book to test the specific primary and/or secondary emotion associated with that gateway and have the client focus on that while you apply one of the many therapies suggested in this book.

Another way with muscle testing is test from the chart to find the imbalanced emotion. Once you find the emotion, you find the associated organ and the appropriate gateway center. When you know the appropriate organ and gateway, you can apply an essential oil to the area on the skin overlying the organ involved and also on the gateway center. This will bring these two parts of the subtle energy system back into communication. While doing this you could place an appropriate stone over the gateway as a combined therapy. Once you have applied one or more of these therapies to the organ and the gateway you can move to the releasing strategy.

Healers that don't use muscle-testing methods or are not allowed to touch their clients:

If you are a healer that does not use muscle-testing methods, you can just have the patient bring their awareness to their body. As they breathe and raise the awareness to their body ask them where the energy feels off, stuck, stagnant or uncomfortable. When you have the area of their body that they have located for you in the process of raising their body awareness you can then use the charts to know what gateway that area is associated with. Once you have the gateway then you can suggest possible emotions that they might be feeling or let them define the emotion themselves. Patients defining the emotion for themselves is more effective because they are pulling it from their own model of the world, their world experience. It is always important to allow them to feel what they feel. Do not try to fit them into a specific emotion. However, whatever the emotion is, you can link where they feel the energy blockage in their body to a specific gateway and apply appropriate therapies based on that.

Regardless of how you get there:

You can proceed by helping them continue to focus their awareness on the emotion they are feeling. Letting them fully experience the emotion. Then, coach them to breathe in fully, keeping their focus on the emotional feeling. As they exhale fully, have them imagine they are fully letting go of the emotion from their body. You will want to repeat this process with as many breaths as is necessary to decrease the energy of the emotion. The emotional intensity may rise when they start this breathing/releasing process but stick with it and then it will start to diminish in intensity. This is how you know the emotional energy pattern is shifting, changing and releasing.

After you feel like the emotion has lost the charged energy it had at the start of the process, you can now lightly tap the gateway center associated with that cleared emotion and with each inhale and exhale that follows, speak the associated mantra or have the client speak it. This is just a reminder phrase that they can express either out loud or quietly inside, depending on their need for or available privacy. The mantra is to return the appropriate energy balance to the gateway and to remind them of the deeper truth about themselves.

If you are inclined or just want to try it out, I recommend that you give them homework after the session and have them utilize one or a combination of the yoga poses associated with that gateway. While in each pose, they can of course, breathe, quietly repeat the mantra, and reflect on how that stuck emotion has impacted their life. This is where we often learn the lesson of why that emotional pattern was in our lives. We can often get additional insights in how that emotion actually served us in some way.

Have fun with this. Explore and enrich your life experience. Breathe. Release tension. Learn. Thrive.

The Seven Gateway Therapies

7th Gateway, the Connection Gateway
Inner and outer beauty, spiritual connection

Chakra: crown

Mantra: "I am a vessel connected to love and light."

Essential oils: frankincense, sandalwood, saffron, lotus, jasmine, lemon, rosewood

Stone: clear quartz

Yoga poses: headstands, half lotus pose, corpse pose

6th Gateway, the Vision Gateway
Intuition, imagination, and wisdom

Chakra: third eye

Mantra: "I am open to peacefully exploring what is not yet clearly seen."

Essential oils: lavender, jasmine, myrrh, patchouli, frankincense, vanilla, frankincense

Stone: amethyst

Yoga poses: shoulder stands, cat/cow pose, child pose

5th Gateway, the Expression Gateway
Communication, self-expression, and truth

Chakra: throat

Mantra: "I express my true self, always."

Essential oils: eucalyptus, rosemary, lemon, sage, cedarwood, lime, German chamomile

Stone: aquamarine

Yoga poses: Shoulder stand, camel pose, plow pose, bridge pose

4th Gateway, the Love Gateway
Love, joy and inner peace

Chakra: heart

Mantra: "When I love myself, and let go of fear, loving others comes easily."

Essential oils: geranium, lime, spearmint, rose, geranium, ylang ylang, jasmine

Stone: rose quartz

Yoga Poses: back bends, eagle pose

3rd Gateway, the Action Gateway
Self-worth, self-confidence, and self-esteem

Chakra: solar plexus

Mantra: "I freely move into action when I accept all parts of myself."

Essential oils: cedarwood, grapefruit, sweet marjoram, fennel, lime, coriander

Stone: amber

Yoga poses: sun salutation, boat pose, leg lifts, mountain pose

2nd Gateway, the Pleasure Gateway
Your sense of abundance, well-being, pleasure and sexuality

Chakra: sacral

Mantra: "I always honor others by honoring myself first."

Essential oils: ylang ylang, sandalwood, jasmine, bergamot, clary sage, neroli

Stone: tiger's eye

Yoga poses: cow face pose, pigeon pose, bond and open angle poses

1st Gateway, the Foundation Gateway

Survival issues such as financial independence, money, food

Chakra: root

Mantra: "I am safe to grow from a steady foundation."

Essential oils: vetiver, myrrh, ginger, rosewood, pine, frankincense, cinnamon

Stone: hematite

Yoga poses: reclining bound angle pose, child pose, forward bend, head to knee pose

I have included some activities that I have discovered in 35 years of practice that will assist you and your patients in processing your Health Code. Acknowledging the language of the body will create clarity on the reasons, perspectives, or beliefs that might be contributing to pain. Once the lesson is learned and the necessary action is understood to return life to a state of balance and harmony, the pain will disappear.

People without these insights or this guide to how energy creates symptoms will do the habitual thing and rush to the medicine cabinet for painkillers. However, those are just numbing tools and the problem will still exist. Some people use other mind/body/life altering things such as alcohol, food, porn, painkillers, or anti-inflammatory drugs and just numb-out. Some veg-out by watching a little more television! Use this section of the book to learn more about establishing communication with the brilliance of the body and be open to new perspectives on pain or life challenges.

Use this section to either work with your clients on their healing or use as homework assignments for them to follow to complete the healings you have initiated with them. Use these concepts to begin the process of retraining your patients as well as your own body-mind to explore and integrate new concepts and perspectives. This will create new options for behavior and give you the ability to begin empowering yourself for constructive thought and positive change in your life. You have also taken an incredibly important step on your life path, one toward growth and away from fear. From this conscious place, you can offer your gifts, talents and inspiration unconditionally to the world.

There are a number of ways for you and your clients to heal the unresolved emotional issues that you discover. By teaching yourself to let go and teaching your patients to let go of the pain in their bodies, you begin the process of letting go in your life and your patients will do the same in their lives. You are consciously releasing emotional baggage and limiting beliefs that we all have been carrying with us. The phrase "letting go" has been overused as a cliché for the last couple of decades. Yet, it is such a powerful inward maneuver that it merits use in our work here. There is much to be learned from the practice of letting go. If you just don't like the phrase "letting go" then at least "let loose" of the stronghold death grip that you have on things. Teach others to "let loose" of those emotions and behaviors that really aren't serving the expression of the best version of themselves at this point.

Letting go means just what it implies. It's giving yourself permission to cease clinging to anything. Whether it is an idea, a thing, an event, a particular time, viewpoint, or desire. To let go means to give up coercing, resisting, or struggling in exchange for something more powerful and peaceful. The power and peacefulness come out of allowing things to be as they are without getting caught up in your attraction to them or rejection of them. Therefore, not getting stuck in the wanting, desiring, liking, or disliking of any particular thing. Letting go is a feeling of freedom—that feeling akin to having worn too tight a pair of shoes all day, and then finally taking them off. AAAHHH!!! Freedom.

Life in its entirety is an epic trek best taken a day at a time. It is like a day hike. If you have ever backpacked for an extended time period, you know you can end up carrying a very heavy pack. We know that life is a long journey. Don't carry from day to day things that don't serve you any longer. Life can be lived day by day, moment by moment. The proper thing to do at the end of each day is unpack.

Before you lie down to sleep, to really rest, choose to let go of whatever baggage has accumulated for that day. When you move through the next day, you will fill your pack once again. At the end of the day, you will empty it again. This way you are able to start the next day without the accumulation of baggage from days, months, or years.

In my practice, I have seen people come with a moving van load of emotional baggage strapped to themselves. They often are carrying the weight of family, job stress, career challenges, financial burdens, and frustrations. Many of these things they have been carrying around for years. Often, they have been carrying family issues since childhood. They are wondering why they have low back pain, shoulder, and neck pain.

The rest of this book is designed to give you some exercises to assist your clients and you to empty your backpack. These tools have come from a wide variety of sources. I have created audio files on all of these processes if you are interested in helpful guidance, with a listing in the reference section of this book. You can use any of these processes separately or in combination with others. Each process stands alone as a powerful tool for change. The idea is to try each of them independently and find the ones that most resonate with you. You can find an application for these processes in any situation or circumstance with which you or your patients are dealing. As you become more familiar with each technique, you will begin to see how combining certain methods can be most powerful for the individual needs of your clients.

Tools Included for Unpacking:

- Breathing (What you need to know)
- Buddha Belly Breathing (The effortless way)
- Breath work (The basics of letting go)
- Visualizations
    * Focused Attention Breathing Visualization
    * Focused Diaphragmatic Breathing (Releasing)
    * Just Relax (A visualization process)
    * Cutting the Strings (Visualization)
    * Energizing the Gateways (Visualization)
- Exercises
    * Body Spotting

* Say It! Love It! Burn It! (Journaling as a tool for transformation)
    * Belief Change Exercise
    * Smashing the Anger (Ice cube therapy)
    * Integrative Tapping
    * STAT (Short Tapas Acupressure Technique)
* Meditations
    * Morning Manifestation Meditation
    * Evening Release Meditation

One thing that is worthy of mention before we continue much further is the difference between emotional reality and historical reality. These may not be familiar concepts to you. Please don't get frustrated or throw in the towel at this point with one more new concept. You have come so far and you're doing really well.

Historical reality is a term used to describe events, memories, situations, or circumstances that actually happened in a person's life—actual verifiable events. For instance, you may remember (when you were five years old) living in a blue house on Pine Street, your room was painted white, and there was a plaid comforter on your bed. These facts can be validated so they are historical. If you had pictures of this room in the family photo album or still had the comforter, you could definitely say this was historical data. You could validate your memory of these things as accurate and real.

Where we actually get into trouble is when we can't historically validate a memory, event, circumstance, story, or picture in our minds. For instance, you may have a memory of being left alone as a small boy at the grocery store by your mother. You may have concluded that this event has given you a lack of trust toward your mother, or women in general. Maybe you claim it is the reason for your feelings of being abandoned. However, you don't have a picture or story from another person's observation to validate this event. This is what is termed emotional reality. The emotion is there even though we don't have evidence of its historical accuracy. In your mother's reality, she may have been one aisle over in the grocery store, picking up a bag of potato chips and returned within moments to your side. The point is whether the emotion is a historical reality or an emotional reality doesn't really matter; what is important is the emotional charge on the event.

When you notice that your client is getting stuck or bogged down in this dilemma, just gently suggest that historical or emotional is not as important as the process of letting go of the emotional charge. If you, or your patient, have charged memories or you are working directly with some issue, don't get hooked on the need to validate it. Otherwise you miss the point of letting go of it. All of these processes are for your benefit and your patients' benefit. The processes are a way to lighten loads and heal lives. Remember, it is the emotional charge that changes physiology. We can assume that if it is charged, it is important. Acknowledge the emotion, align with the desire to be done with it, let go of it, and let the Universe/God/Nature/whatever your name is for the source of all knowing, work out the details.

Michelangelo's genius as a sculptor lay in his ability to see a finished statue inside a rough block of marble. His challenge was not to make a sculpture, but to release the one that was already there, imprisoned in the stone. Your challenge in using the following processes is the same. You, nor your patients, are creating new identities; you and your clients are releasing the potential found within each of you. You, or your patients, will be releasing the best and most perfect version of yourselves that already exist and have always been inside. The process is one of self-discovery. I believe there is one extremely important process that must be re-learned or remembered before much else can happen and anyone, especially your clients, begins self-improvement or self-healing. It is not mandatory for doing any of these processes, yet it is beneficial. That one extremely important process is breathing. I could talk for days on end about breathing. It is the basis of many yoga, meditation, prayer, and relaxation methods. Ancient Vedic texts, the Bible, Hindu, Muslim, Buddhist, and other recent texts all refer to the art of breathing. We have all been doing it for years and have probably not given it much thought. Well, I'm asking you to look at breathing as if you have never seen it before or experienced it before. I'm asking you to slow down and teach anyone you work with to breathe. I'm asking you not to jump past this part in the next section on visualizations, exercises and meditations. You may say, "That's stupid, I already know how to breathe. Why do I need to learn about breathing?" I promise I'll keep these steps short and sweet, yet powerful for you.

Awareness Keys

- You can begin to see that symptoms you or your clients experience in your bodies can give you insights into the underlying emotions that are part of the problem.

- It is healthy to listen to gentle whispers of these emotions before the body resorts to shouting by way of symptoms.

- The subtle energy systems, the bio-emotional gateways, acupuncture, chakra and nervous systems are interrelated.

- In the charts, each organ and its related meridian channel are associated with a gateway and chakra center.

- Utilizing the seven gateway therapies is an effective way to release emotions from the subtle energy systems and symptoms from the body.

- Teaching yourself and your patients to acknowledge the language of your body, the Health Code, will create clarity on what is contributing to your pain.

- Letting go means giving yourself permission to stop clinging to anything. Whether it's an idea, a thing, an event, a particular time, viewpoint or desire.

- Unload your daily backpack and teach your clients to unload their backpacks of emotional stuff. Before you lie down to sleep, to really rest, choose to let go of whatever baggage has accumulated for that day.

Chapter 13

Visualizations, Exercises, and Meditations

You can use these methods for your own healing and personal growth, which I recommend since we know that as healers, we must do the work to be the best possible version of a healer. The more we clear our own energy blocks, the more we can serve others as a clean conduit of healing light. All of these methods and exercises can be used with clients as a healing process on their own, or in combination with whatever therapy you already perform in your healing practice. You can combine some of these methods together for a deeper or more specific healing process for your clients. Let your intuition guide you in how best to incorporate these methods into your healing practice.

Breathing

Breathing is a natural phenomenon that we all experience throughout the day. If you weren't breathing, you wouldn't be reading this book. The problem is not that we don't breathe. More accurately, the problem is that we don't breathe efficiently. Whenever we are startled, traumatized, are afraid, or anxious, we alter our pattern of breathing. We shift the center of our breathing from the abdomen to the chest. We still have air going in and out, but the volume and quality of oxygen-filled air is diminished. This decreased quality and quantity of oxygen has a negative impact on our physiology. It impacts the way our body performs its daily functions.

The place where we hold tightly to our emotions is the solar plexus, where the abdomen, ribs, and diaphragm meet. Breathing properly brings air, muscular movement, and attention to the solar plexus. This causes a natural release of stored emotional energy from the body.

The stressful environment of contemporary life has led to the habit of rapid, irregular breathing that takes place predominantly in the upper chest. This breathing pattern stresses the heart, accounts for lower oxygenation of the blood, and limits blood flow. These changes accentuate the accumulation of toxins in the soft tissues, and tend to keep us emotionally, not to mention physically, stressed. We can reduce this stress through diaphragmatic breathing or, as it is affectionately called in my office, Buddha Belly Breathing.

Deep Buddha Belly Breathing provides a number of health benefits. Deep breathing brings more air to the lower lobes of the lungs, which are more richly supplied with blood vessels. This means the blood can absorb more oxygen. Deep breathing lowers pressure within the chest cavity, thereby improving blood circulation, making it easier for blood to return to the heart. This reduces stress and the load on the heart.

Continuous deep breathing generates considerable energy, which when utilized in a positive manner, can improve your focus, stamina, and (best of all) the quality of your sexual experience. If this energy is not utilized positively or is blocked from being expressed, it gets concentrated in areas of the body and causes tension. These blocked or stagnant areas may then store repressed images, feelings, or emotional trauma. These repressed energies often create discomfort or pain in the body until they are released.

Buddha Belly Breathing (Diaphragmatic Breathing)

- Sit on the forward edge of a comfortable chair and lean back so that you are slightly reclining or lie on your back on the floor with your knees up in a comfortable position.

- Place one hand palm down over your navel. Place the other hand palm down on the center of your chest.

- Exhale completely to start, releasing as much air out of your lungs as possible, as if breathing a sigh of relief.

- Next, draw your breath inward while imagining that your abdomen is expanding like a balloon. Hence, a Buddha belly—round, expanded, and relaxed, like the statues of Buddha you may have seen. Notice that your abdomen is expanding more than your chest.

  **Note: If you don't get this at first, it's okay. Many of us have forgotten the proper way of breathing since we were newborn babies. This is truly how we breathe when we are newly born, but over time we learn or are trained out of this natural process. When we find ourselves having to relearn or retrain ourselves, it is just a diagnostic sign to yourself that you need to practice this exercise even more often until you can accomplish it naturally.

- As you exhale, imagine this balloon deflating and flattening.

After 10 to 12 diaphragmatic breaths, become aware of how you feel. Is your body more relaxed? Is your mind calmer? Do you feel more at peace? Often people experience one, if not all three, of these feelings.

Now you have a clue about the proper method of breathing. I suggest you practice this method daily, and especially when stressful situations present themselves in your daily activities. It will be to your advantage to use this type of breathing while doing the processes that follow in this book. Let go, have fun, create positive energy, and heal.

Breath Work (The Basics of Letting Go)

Breathing is often taken for granted. Breath is life. Spiritus is the Latin word for breath, meaning the animating or vital principle that gives life to physical organisms. English words for breath reflect this origin in respiration, inspiration, and expiration. The Chinese word Chi has a similar dual meaning of "life" and "breath." Sanskrit expresses the life force as "prana." The yogis have been exploring the relationship between breathing and consciousness for more than two thousand years. I have found breath work to be the most powerful tool for transformation that we can utilize. Besides, it's always there, it doesn't cost anything, and it works incredibly well at releasing unresolved emotion from the body.

With proper use of breathing, you can literally transform stuck, unresolved emotion into pure energy. The transformation occurs in several ways:

- Breath work brings awareness to an area of the body where emotions are stored, stuck, or just plain hangin' out and causing havoc.

- Breath work releases the unresolved emotions from the cells, tissues, and organs of the body.

- Breath work can release old birth trauma or shock from previous traumatic events, things we were not processing that were stored away in the body at a very early time in our lives.

- Breath work can alter physiology and profoundly affect the autonomic nervous system, the impact of which can alter discomfort in the body, chronic pain, or overall physiological wellness.

- Breath work can open the doorway to other-than-conscious emotional baggage, memories, or trauma that show up as persistent repeating life patterns that may not be serving our higher good any longer. I think they call this self-sabotage.

- Breath work increases the amount of positive energy you can inhale. It keeps your heart center open to allow what you are experiencing moment to moment to flow through you.

- Breath work brings you to profound interactive relationship with the Infinitely Intelligent Self, the Sacred Self, and keeps the flow through all of the bioemotional gateways.

It is vital in breath work of any type to keep awareness open and love flowing. Love is the healing energy that will move pain, trauma, and unresolved emotions. There are experiences and issues that will only be healed by love, acceptance, and forgiveness. Let's begin. Let's move into healing.

Visualizations

Focused Attention Breathing Visualization

You may want to preface this Focused Attention Visualization process with the Just Relax Visualization to allow a deeper level of tuning into your body. However, this process can stand on its own without doing the Just Relax Visualization first. Once in a relaxed state, begin to notice an area of pain, tension, injury, or discomfort in your body. Bring your attention and awareness to that area. Notice what shape it takes. Notice what color it is. Notice what thought, feeling, or emotion it has.

Now, give it a voice and let it tell you what purpose it serves. Let it tell you what lesson it is there to teach you. Ask it questions if you like. Tell it you are here to honor its presence and want to learn from it. What does it need to tell you about your life, so that it can let go and know you have gotten the message?

If it feels safe and you want to, mentally step inside of this shape or space. Notice where you are once inside of it. Let a guide, a special person, or friend come to you in this space. Once this guide or person appears to you, question them about this pain, discomfort, or trauma. Listen to what they have to say to you. Be open and curious to this teaching, or information, and see how it applies to your life or your current life situation.

Thank that person or guide for helping you with your understanding of the lesson associated with this pain. Allow your awareness to come out of the shape. Now, allow your mind to transform this shape into something beautiful, a symbol of change, or a symbol of letting go.

Return your attention to your breathing and to your heartbeat. Love yourself. Love the area where your discomfort was. Let go of anything that is still lingering in that area.

Let yourself begin to feel your surroundings. Notice how your lips and face feel. Be aware of the energy returning to your feet and hands. Let your awareness completely return to this present time, returning now, fully awake and at peace, and remembering all the lessons you received.

Breathe and relax and be present.

Focused Diaphragmatic Breathing (Releasing)

Now using Focused-Attention Breathing from an earlier exercise, we are going to combine this with the Buddha Belly Breathing from earlier.

- Lie down, flat or knees bent. Eyes may be open or closed. Be comfortable. Loosen your belt or any constricting clothing as needed.

- Look through your mind's eye into your body for areas of pain or discomfort. If there is no area of pain look for areas of stuck or stagnant energy in the body. Review expectations, intentions, or goals that have constricted energy or limitation around them. Look for fears that are keeping you from moving forward in your life.

- Open your throat by slightly tilting your head back. Relax your jaws and throat muscles. Breathe in and out through an open mouth to start; this keeps the throat open and relaxed. If the throat is relaxed and free, then energy flows through the whole person.

- Relax the throat and breathe so that you can say AAHHH. When the sound is open, deep, clear, and full it indicates that energy is flowing through the body in an optimum way. If it is shallow, ragged, or hesitant, it means you are wrestling with a block or suppressed emotion. It is important to get the throat open and flowing because as energy and breath move through your body there will be other areas opening. This energy will need to be released through the throat. Now, breathe in and out with a silent AAHHH.

- Begin the breathing process. Pace the process as fast or as slow as you wish. Establish a rhythm and be sensitive to it wanting to change pace. If you sense that you are breathing slowly to avoid feeling something, I encourage you to speed up. If you are breathing fast to avoid feeling something, I encourage you to slow down.

- Take each experience as it comes. Accept and flow with whatever emerges. Most of the good things appear when you let go of control, when you stop resisting. Let go just a little bit. Let go of your judgment ("Is this the experience I'm supposed to be having?") and simply take things as they come. Stay open and curious. I invite you to adopt a body attitude of openness and willingness by relaxing the throat and breathing fully in and out.

- If you feel like you have lost the form, are struggling with taking a full open breath, or lose awareness, it's okay. Simply notice you have lost it and return to it. Don't force it or make it work, relax into it.

- Pleasant and unpleasant feelings may emerge. All feelings turn into positive energy if experienced fully. When we are fully open, the range of emotions from rage to bliss come out of the same faucet. Our only decision is whether or not to open the faucet. Our choice can be to experience the complete spectrum of emotions and generate positive energy from there. If during this breathing exercise your body wants to spontaneously move in some way, try allowing this movement and keep breathing. This may be the nervous system "shaking it off." Remember that shaking and unwinding of the tissues of the body may be the release of stored emotions or trauma. Let the intelligence of the body and mind do what they need to do.

- Stop when you feel peace or bliss, or when you have come to a peaceful stopping place that is free from fear. Never stop in the midst of a block or when you are feeling bad for any reason. Always breathe through it. If you feel like you want to stop, ask yourself if you are feeling any fear or unpleasantness in your body. If so, continue breathing until it passes before stopping. Oddly enough, humans have as much resistance to positive energy as they do to negative. Most people will say that they prefer bliss and pleasurable experiences to painful ones. In the breath work I have done, I have found this not to be true. I have experienced people sobbing for an hour, sometimes in waves for an entire day. I have yet to experience a person who can sustain more than five minutes of ecstasy or bliss. Most of us have hundreds of hours of experiencing negative energy. We are still learning to crawl when it comes to feeling good, feeling positive, and being able to sustain bliss.

The reason most of us can't sustain highs and lows in our lives is because we operate within a comfort zone of our feeling experience. It is described and defined well by Gay and Kathleen Hendricks from the Hendricks Institute, as the Upper Limits Problem. In brief, it means that we tend to operate emotionally in a comfort zone. If we have too high an emotional experience, we will automatically correct ourselves from our subconscious mind to return into our comfort zone. It also works the opposite way. If we go too far below our comfort zone, we will automatically correct to raise ourselves back up into our comfort zone. We do this by sabotaging our experiences in life in simple yet effective ways even though they may be destructive to our growth.

Often, if we are having a wonderful connection in our relationship with our partner, we will feel really good, connected, and passionate. If this pushes us out of our comfort zone, we will notice that we unconsciously begin to nitpick their behavior, or we get irritated and pick a fight or a quarrel over something minor. This allows us to move out of our upper limit of feeling and experiencing the bliss of our relationship and brings us back to our comfort zone. Why would we do this? Well, we just can't seem to sustain that feeling of continuous growth and enjoyment of the experience. The same happens at the bottom of the wave as well. If we are too low and out of our comfort zone, we will find experiences to help us find our way back into to a better place within our comfort zone. This doesn't seem unreasonable at all. And it isn't—unless, we are using destructive behavior to get us there.

There is a lot to be said about this; however, that is not the topic of this book.

Just Relax Visualization

One of the best ways to begin the process of letting go and allowing your body to become more energetic, lighter, and more flexible is to train the body to relax at a very deep level. Often times, if practiced enough, you can train your body to relax at a moment's notice. By returning to a relaxed breathing rhythm and by visualizing a specific predesigned anchor or stimulus, you can obtain a relaxation response quickly. So, let's give it a try.

You can have someone read this to you while you follow along or you can read this section into a digital recorder and play it back to yourself. Another option is you may want to download it from my website where I have prepared it, combining background music and voice for a convenient relaxing experience.

To begin, find a comfortable and warm place that feels safe. You want to make sure that you will not be disturbed for approximately 30 minutes. You may want to lie down; however, sitting up is fine as well. Begin with a slow, easy, breathing pace. Breathe in slowly, and then out slowly. In through your nose, and out through your mouth. Let your body relax into the rhythm of your breathing.

As you continue to breathe in and out slowly, imagine there is a glowing ball of light energy at your feet. Let it be a nurturing light with a pleasant color, maybe your favorite color. As you inhale, allow this light, this colored energy, to enter the soles of your feet, slowly moving into your feet and ankles. Then slowly, with each breath, let the color move to your calves, filling the entire calf. Allow this color, energy, to move through your knees, letting your knees, calves, ankles, and feet relax.

With each rhythmic breath, let the light, soft, color float up through your thighs and hips. Letting it move into your buttocks and pour over your hips, into your pelvis. Let all of the muscles, ligaments, and tendons relax. As you breathe, notice that your pelvis and lower abdomen begin to fill with this loving color. Let your stomach, low back, and pelvis relax completely. Allow the area below your diaphragm to fill with this relaxing, soothing, nurturing, color and let the large intestine, stomach, liver, pancreas, and spleen relax. Let your kidneys, gallbladder, and spine relax.

As you inhale, let the softness of the color penetrate through the diaphragm, letting all the tightness in the solar plexus relax. As you relax, let the emotional tightness and energy release from this area and the lower half of your body. Notice the color moving, now into your chest, filling your lungs, surrounding your heart, and softening all the hurt and painful issues that keep you from unconditionally loving yourself and others. Let the color and relaxation move into your shoulders and down your arms, flowing into your elbows, forearms, wrists, and hands. Let your shoulders, arms, hands, and fingers totally relax. Allow color to fill your neck area, front and back, relaxing your voice and the muscles of the back of your neck.

Move the soft, relaxing color up to your jaws and cheeks, warming the muscles, releasing tension and melting into relaxation. Empty your forehead of all tension there, let your face relax, even relax your lips. Now let go of the tension in your scalp and let the color fill your head. Silence your mind and feel your breath. Feel the movement of color through your body, breathing in and out slowly.

Now let your focus and attention be on your heart area, the center of your chest. Feel the vibration beating there, the rhythm. Imagine now that there is energy spiraling around your heart. Notice that the spirals begin to extend down from your heart, flowing through your body all the way to your feet. Also notice that the energy spirals upward from your heart through your body all the way to the very top of your head.

Feel the energy and notice whether it is constricted or expansive. Allow it to be expansive, generous, and open. Let this energy be unconditional love for yourself and for all living things in the Universe. Let the spirals expand into wider rings of energy. Let the spirals expand out to the edges of your body. Feel the love, peace, and harmony of this energy. Let this energy expand out of you and into the space you occupy right now. Let the energy expand down through the earth and out into the Universe. Let the energy encompass the entire planet.

Send this loving and radiant energy to anyone you wish to touch, heal, forgive, or nurture. Think or create an image of that person in your mind. See yourself sending this energy to them from the place you are in right now. Then let the image of them go. Find another person and do the same. Take a few minutes and just touch others with this energy. Now begin to bring this expansive energy back to your heart center, let the movement of the spirals continue with each breath and each beat of your heart. Feel the freshness of this energy and allow that energy to stay expansive, light, and peaceful as you begin to notice each breath, in and out. Let yourself bathe in the unconditional energy of the Universe, be grateful for the presence of this energy around you and within you. Now, begin to notice the sounds around you and notice the feeling in your lips, feet and hands. Notice the warm feeling inside your body and notice the feeling in your arms, hands, legs, and hips. As you awaken, return energized, peaceful, and balanced from this journey. Come totally back to this time and space, bringing yourself back to the present now.

Cutting the Strings Visualization

This visualization can begin by doing the Just Relax Visualization first. Rather than coming out of the Just Relax Visualization, continue if you like with the Cutting the Strings Visualization that follows. It is perfectly fine to do Cutting the Strings Visualization all by itself as well. One powerful pattern is to start with Cutting the Strings and then finish with Just Relax Visualization.

Let's focus your attention on a certain area of your physical body where there has been some pain or muscle tightness. Take a moment and just check on that area and see what images appear in your mind's eye. What shape is the pain or discomfort? What color is it? What is the texture of it? Notice if it has a thought, feeling, or emotion with it. If so, when you experience that thought, feeling, or emotion, how old do you feel? What was going on for you at that age? Is there a specific incident, event, or person that is associated with or appears in this image? If so, who? As hard as it may be to consider doing, does this person, event, or circumstance, need to be forgiven?

Remember, when forgiving someone that does not mean you forgive their behavior. Forgiveness is a gift for yourself, to allow yourself to let go of the hurt and trauma of the event. Forgiveness is for your benefit and your freedom from the feelings. If you can bring yourself to forgive this person, then bring that person or event more into focus. Have that person appear a safe distance away, but in front of you, now.

Take a moment and tell that person everything you have ever wanted to tell them, but haven't or didn't about your pain around the event or circumstance. Take a few minutes and really feel the emotion. Let it out, whatever you need to say. This is the time to do it, in the privacy of your own mind, room, or quiet place.

For now, finish this process of letting it out. Keep the person or event in front of you. If you feel at this time that you can do this, tell them that you love them and forgive them. Now, I understand that this might not be possible. So, if you can't even get close to forgiveness, then say, "I'm willing to consider the possibility of loving you and forgiving you at some time in the future." That will work and is fine as well. Remember, you are loving and forgiving the humanness of this being, not their behavior. It is possible to love the person and not like the behavior they exhibit.

Now tell yourself that you love yourself and forgive yourself for carrying this memory or unloving, stagnate energy around in your cosmic backpack, in your body, mind, heart, and spirit. Be generous to yourself. Take a moment to appreciate the loving, precious, peaceful being that you are in your true nature. Give thanks for the talents and gifts that you possess and that you so graciously bring to this life.

Once again, look at the person before you; notice that there are connections, cords, coming from the person to you. At this time, I ask you to cut the cords, making sure all of the cords are cut away from you and separated from you now, forever. These cords are connections of dissonant, disruptive energy between the two of you. In this moment, tell this person that you want them to give your power back to you regardless if you gave your power away to them, or you feel they took your power from you. You want it back in full. So, have them put your power into a gift box and wrap it up in beautiful packaging, maybe even with a bow. Then place it in front of you.

When you have cut all the cords and have your gift in front of you, surround the person in a pink, light, airy bubble. Using the steps below, take three deep, slow breaths, in through your nose and out through your mouth. As you do this, blow the pink bubble further and further away from you with each breath.

- First inhale. Now blow out and watch the bubble drift out of the place where you are currently.

- Second, inhale and exhale again, blowing the bubble into the clouds or the blue of the sky.

- Now third, breathe in and blow out, blowing the bubble way out into the Universe and, POP! Let the bubble burst and be gone, forever.

Settle your breathing and let your body relax. Notice the gift in front of you. Open it. Notice that there is a symbol of your power inside. What is that symbol? Now, take your symbol and your power into your hands again. Hold it and feel it. Feel the energy of it. Then gently take the symbol and place it in your heart, never to be given away or taken away again.

Scan your body now to see if there are any empty, blank, or dark spaces in your body where you have let go of limiting or trapped emotions, images, or memories. If so, fill these areas with a bright, radiant white light. Pull that light inside, asking it to fill up the dark empty spaces with love, life, laughter, and grace.

See the light filing up these spaces now. See them sparkling with healing, nurturing, and energizing light. Imagine it's much like the sight of early morning sunlight caressing the vastness of the ocean as you walk on a beach, or caressing a fresh, crisp, winter snow-fall sparkling and clear. Now breathe in this new, light, relaxed way of being.

Begin to notice your breathing again. Begin to notice your body, stretch your feet and legs, feel your lips and notice your surroundings. Breathing slowly and rhythmically, allow yourself to come totally back, energized, light, filled with love, peace, and harmony. Come all the way back and be present where you are, now.

Energizing the Gateways Visualization

This is a powerful visualization for energizing all seven gateways in your body. It is an awesome way to clear the gateways and to also flush out any stuck energy in the system that may have slipped through during your busy schedule. Clients have reported that doing this visualization has been extremely effective in helping them keep their overall energy high. A consistent practice of this visualization can help increase immune function and also energize as well as clear the organ systems associated with each bioemotional gateway, chakra, and nerve plexus.

The Method:

- Find a safe and relaxed place to be able to sit or lie down.

- Make sure you won't be interrupted for about 20 – 30 minutes.

- Close your eyes and begin to slowly and methodically deep breathe in and out.

- Bring your focus to the First Gateway at the floor of the pelvis and inhaling with the intention to draw your inner energy up through your body to the Seventh Gateway at the crown of your head. Allow this energy to move through you for a few rounds of breathing.

- Slowly begin to put your attention on each Gateway tuned into any stress, discomfort, or other sensation that is in each Gateway area.

- Start to repeat in your mind at the different Gateways the healing phrase listed below and notice what surfaces to be experienced. Just continue to breathe through the disruption and notice when the feeling starts to dissipate. At the point where the negative energy starts to fade, you can repeat the healing phrase one more time; then move to the next Gateway and begin the same process moving through each of the 7 Gateways using the healing phrase for that Healing Gateway.

- Foundation Gateway #1 phrase: "I am safe to grow from a steady foundation."

- Pleasure Gateway #2 phrase: "I always honor others by honoring myself first."

- Action Gateway #3 phrase: "I freely move into action when I accept all parts of myself. "

- Love Gateway #4 phrase: "When I love myself and let go of fear, loving others comes easily."

- Expression Gateway #5 phrase: "I express my true self, always."

- Vision Gateway #6 phrase: "I am open to peacefully exploring what is not yet clearly seen."

- Connection Gateway #7 phrase: "I am a vessel connected to love and light."

At the end of the visualization, I recommend mentally focusing on each of the gateways starting at the crown and moving through the foundation/root, stating each of the phrases in one continuous flow to complete the full cycle of energy through the centers. Slowly open your eyes and go about your day.

You may want to journal about what thoughts or experiences presented themselves during your process. You might want to journal about what epiphanies come to you and about what these thoughts or experiences are trying to teach you.

Exercises

Body Spotting Method

This visualization can be done daily as a means of finding where you are holding stored emotional energy or emotional trauma from day to day. As you move through any day of activity, you may get triggered from some old past event or trauma. That trigger may bring emotional baggage up to the surface and create an opportunity to release old limiting behavior patterns. So, this can be valuable to your ultimate freedom and happiness in life.

- You may want to preface this visualization process with Just Relax Visualization to allow a deeper level of synchronization with your body. However, this process can stand on its own without doing the Just Relax Visualization first.

- Once in a relaxed state, begin to notice an area of pain, tension, injury, or discomfort in your body. Bring your attention and awareness to that area.

- Notice what shape it takes. Perhaps it is more circular, triangular, square, oval, starburst, etc.

- Notice what color it is.

- Notice the texture of the area, rough, smooth, chaotic, flowing.

- Notice the temperature of this region, hot, cold, tepid, freezing.

- Let your breath carry your awareness into this colored shape and allow your awareness to just sit inside this area. Notice what thought, feeling, or emotion is present inside this area.

- Allow yourself to inhale and feel that emotion, thought, or feeling and as you exhale, allow yourself to let go of that thought, feeling, or emotion.

- Breathe in again feeling that thought, feeling, or emotion and breathe out to let it go again. Repeat this breathing process till you notice that the thought, feeling, or emotion is fading away.

- When it feels like the thought, feeling, or emotion is fading away, take two more breaths and be willing to let go of whatever residual feeling is there.

- Now, notice what thought, feeling, or emotion is right underneath the last feeling.

- Once you identify that underlying thought, feeling, or emotion, repeat this process until you feel a sense of peace, calm, or a smile emerges spontaneously on your face.

Say it! Love it! Burn it!
(Journaling as a tool for transformation)

Journaling is a profound way to physically move the energy of unresolved emotional issues that are stuck in your physiology (body). I have discovered in practice that often during a journaling process you will have emotions emerge in the form of crying, sadness, anger, rage, or nausea. You may need to take a break from time to time and return to the breath work exercise (the basics of letting go) or more specifically, Focused Diaphragmatic Breathing (release) in order to properly process emotions that do arise. If you skipped that part of this book then naughty, naughty. It would be very beneficial for you to go review that exercise as well as breathing and breath work so that you can get the most powerful effect from this exercise and be best equipped to handle the emotional release.

I devised this journaling process thirty years ago and have had thousands of clients use it over time. It is an extremely powerful and transformative process if you truly let go and let it come through you, so to speak. Holding back is not being generous to yourself.

Let it rip, you'll get more out of it. Besides, you're not going to send it; you're going to burn it. So, who's going to find out?

Here is how it goes. The following letter can be written to anyone with whom you feel there are issues that remain unresolved or with whom you have an issue or there exists any negative energy. It can even be written to an aspect of yourself; address the letter to your critical self, judgmental self, or that doubting voice inside.

Below is a sample letter that you can reproduce and use for as many people, situations, or parts of yourself as you wish. Feel free to be free and write your own pure content, too. Good luck; don't hold anything back and have a great process.

Dear _____,

[Tell this person, part of yourself or situation everything you have ever wanted to tell them, but you haven't or didn't. You are not going to send this letter, so be willing to let it rip.]

(I highly recommend under no circumstances should you actually send this letter, even if you feel it is justifiable to do so.)

In the process of writing this letter you may experience a variety of emotions coming up for you, such as rage, fear, anger, sadness or even guilt. Take time to fully feel them and keep writing.

You may want to include the feelings in your journaling process so that you can identify the energy that has been festering inside you.

You may complete this letter in a mere paragraph, or it may take you 15 pages. Whatever it takes, just stay with it. It will pay off in the long run.

When you feel you have written and expressed all there is to express, then write at the end of the letter and write with intention:

I love you and forgive you.
I love myself and forgive myself for
- Carrying this around in my body
- My part in creating this in my life
- Holding on to the energy of this in my mind, body and spirit.

Pick one of the appropriate endings for your situation or make up your own.

If for some reason you are unable to carry out the above process, get as close to it as you possibly can. For instance, you could write: I'm willing to consider the possibility of loving and forgiving you at some time in the future. Hey, I know we are really hedging here, but sometimes that's as close as we can get especially with emotions that are festering for years and creating dysfunction for you. So, go with it and feel good.

Then, finish the letter with this powerful affirmation:

I release all constricted energy between us now and I claim that energy back for my complete mental, emotional, spiritual, and physical healing. I do this through love and with love. I invite back to me only peace, love, prosperity, and the greatness that is my inheritance from my Source. I live each day in expectancy of this or something even better.

Then, create a ceremony in which your central theme is to burn the letter, allowing the smoke from the burning pages to lift the burden of the letter up to your angels, guides, God, or your Source. At the end of the bonfire (just kidding), either stomp on the ashes or bury them.

In approximately 10 – 14 days you will receive a sign from the Universe or your Source that the energy around this situation, event, or person has changed and is cleared. Only you will recognize the sign. I've seen amazing things and amazing healings occur with this letter process. So, open your mind and heart and go for the gusto!

Beliefs Change Exercise

How Do Beliefs Work:

The only way to change your beliefs and perceptions in order to create a new life story is to change your state of being. You have to finally see your old, limited beliefs for what they are—records of the past—and be willing to let go of them so that you can embrace new beliefs about yourself that will help you create a new future.

Let's consider what things we could do or ways we could generate to support letting go of our limiting belief statements and integrating our new beliefs. We are currently living from unconscious belief statements. If we want to change, we have to define our new belief statements, try them on and live into them.

My colleague and brain research mentor, Dr. Joe Dispenza puts the concepts of this process into a meticulously researched explanation in all of his books and lectures. In the next few paragraphs you will find my distillation of those concepts as they pertain to this book and this exercise. I offer up love and deep gratitude to Dr. Joe Dispenza for his work and his research.

You see, there are thoughts, feelings, attitudes, beliefs, and perceptions. When you string a succession of thoughts and feelings together so that they ultimately become habituated or automatic, they form an attitude. And since how you think and feel creates a state of being, attitudes are really just extended states of being. They can fluctuate from moment to moment as you alter how you think and feel. Any particular attitude can last for minutes, hours, days, or even a week or two.

Example: if you have a series of good thoughts that are aligned with a series of good feelings, you might say, "I have a good attitude today." If you have a sequence of negative thoughts that are connected to a sequence of negative feelings, then you might say, "I have a bad attitude today." If you revisit the same attitude enough times, then it becomes automatic or habitual.

If you repeat or maintain certain attitudes long enough and you string those attitudes together that is how you create a belief. A belief is just an extended state of being. Essentially, beliefs are thoughts and feelings that have become attitudes that you keep thinking and feeling over and over again until you hardwire them in your brain and emotionally condition them into your body. Because experiences are neurologically etched into your brain (causing you to think) and chemically etched into our bodies as emotions (causing you to feel), your beliefs are based on past thoughts and feelings that generate the same attitudes. You could say that you become addicted to your beliefs, which is why it's so hard to change them and why it doesn't feel good on a gut level when they're challenged.

When you think the same thoughts and feel the same feelings, you experience the same emotions over and over. This cycle of thinking and feeling, feeling and thinking will "fire and wire" into an automatic unconscious program. If you experience the same feelings based on past experiences and experience the same emotions, you'll condition your body to subconsciously be the "mind" of that emotion. Therefore, your body will unconsciously be chemically or physiologically living in the past. This is why I approach healing and the Health Code from the aspect of emotions. This is why bottom-up thinking is important. We can approach healing from the mind, our thinking, and that works well. However, a combination of healing from the language of the body (emotions) and from our mind may be best. I feel this body-mind perspective gives us more access to clear out all of our systems and rewire our brains at the same time.

If the redundancy of how you think and feel over time conditions your body to become the mind and it becomes programmed subconsciously, then beliefs are just the body-mind experiencing unconscious states of being derived from the past. Beliefs are also more permanent than attitudes; they can last for months or even years. And because they last longer, they become more programmed within you.

If you string a group of related beliefs together, they form your perception. Your perception of reality is a sustained state of being that's based on your long-standing beliefs, attitudes, thoughts, and feelings. It's why people say perception is reality.

What follows then is that scientific experiments have shown that you don't see reality as it truly is. Instead, you unconsciously fill in your reality based on your memories of the past, your perceptions. These are a string of beliefs that are neurologically maintained in your brain and chemically maintained in your body. When perceptions become implicit, meaning unquestioned or absolute, they become automatic and you edit reality subjectively. Research has shown that fifty percent of our reality is literally made up. Wow!

Now, if you want to change an implicit or subconscious perception, you must become more conscious about doing so, and not allow your programmed unconscious to run you down the rails. In truth, you have to wake up and consciously decide what you want to believe and create a strategy to rewire your neurology.

But it's rarely that easy, because if you experience the same crafted reality over and over again, then the way you think and feel about your current world will continue to develop into the same attitudes, which will inspire the same beliefs, which will expand into the same perceptions.

When we decide how we want our lives to be, we then have a blueprint for designing the strategies to get us there. Strategies are just the many different ways we generate to get us to the best life possible. These established strategies work backward from perceptions to beliefs to unravel the ideas that perpetuate your perceptions. Once there, you can then look at what attitude you need to have to support a specific belief and what thoughts and feelings you would need to maintain that attitude. You see, you are back at a state but a consciously selected state with improvements in your energy flow and how you see your situation. Next to develop would be what stories would you want to create, where you can think and talk to yourself (or others) that support the new changes. Let's get started.

Changing your beliefs:

Once at this step, ask yourself what beliefs and perceptions about yourself and your life have you been unconsciously agreeing to that you'd have to change in order to create this new state of being? This is a question that requires some thought, because, as I said with many of these beliefs, we aren't even aware that we believe them.

Often, we accept certain cues from our environment that then prime us to accept certain beliefs, which may or may not be true. Whichever way, the moment we accept the belief, it has an effect not only on our performance, but also on the choices we make. The most important statements for which you will become aligned are those that matter most to YOU! These are part of the rhythm of your true self-expression and this is why it's important to define a compelling belief statement.

That said, decide in this moment, "what do you believe now, that isn't working for you?" Maybe it is, "People don't appreciate me," or "Others don't value my skill, talent, ability, and contribution." Maybe, it is, "I'm not worthy of making the money I want or need," or "I'm not good enough, pretty enough, smart enough." These are what are called limiting beliefs. They limit your potential and your possibilities.

So, what are the beliefs that are playing for you now, ones that are getting in the way of you being the best version of yourself? You may want to start to list them. Write down as many as you can think of. (We can pick one to use later). To help you better understand this concept of limiting beliefs let's expand more on this for you.

Limiting Beliefs

In general, there are four different types of limiting beliefs. As you read through the following types, you may begin to identify some of your own unconscious limiting beliefs.

Get a piece of paper and divide it down the middle of the page from top to bottom. On the left side begin a list as directed below:

1. Beliefs about cause. These are beliefs where you believe that there is a specific cause creating the belief. Often these beliefs have the word 'because' in them. Some examples of limiting beliefs about cause include:

- I can't be successful because my parents weren't successful.
- I don't deserve to have what I want because I'm a woman.
- Life is a struggle because I never get what I want.
- We're not supposed to have money because we grew up poor.
- Money causes pain.
- Being successful will cause the family to split.

Write down any beliefs about cause that apply directly to you on the left side of this paper.

2. Beliefs about meaning. As human beings, we are always trying to find the meanings in things. For example, what does it really mean to be rich or poor? What is the deeper meaning behind money? The meanings that you put on these beliefs will guide your behavior because they operate as filters for your belief systems. Some limiting beliefs about meaning include:

- Money doesn't buy happiness.
- Money is the root of all evil.
- Having money isn't spiritual.
- Money is unimportant.
- Earning money would be boring.
- You can't trust rich people.

Write down any beliefs about meaning that apply directly to you on the left side of this paper

3. Beliefs about possibility. Beliefs can also be about possibility and what is possible for us. There are two kinds of beliefs about possibility:

a. The outcome is possible: If it is possible, then you have permission from your subconscious mind to go for the intended goal or outcome.

b. The outcome is impossible: If it is impossible, then you won't even bother trying to get what you want. For example, if you believe that you can't get ahead because the economy is bad and you hold that belief firmly in your mind, then you won't do what it takes to be successful. You will give up ahead of time and not do anything to create what you want.

Some examples of limiting beliefs and possibility include:

- Money is hard to manage; I will never be able to manage money.
- I don't know how to change my life.
- I will never get what I want in life.
- I will never make a lot of money.
- If I make money, I will mess it up and lose it all.

Write down any beliefs about possibility that apply directly to you on the left side of this paper.

4. Identify. Beliefs that involve identity are about our worthiness and deservedness to attain what we want in life, with wealth, regarding happiness, around fulfillment, and achieving success. Some examples of these kinds of limiting beliefs include:

- I am not good enough to be successful.
- I don't deserve to have what I want.
- I am not smart enough to make money.
- I don't know enough to be successful.
- I am not worthy of having life the way I want it.

Write down any beliefs about identity that apply directly to you on the left side of this paper.

The most common unconscious belief issues tend to fall into one or more of the following three categories:

HOPELESSNESS: Belief that the desired goal is not achievable, regardless of your capabilities. There is no hope that you will get what you want.

HELPLESSNESS: Belief that the desired goal is possible, but you are not capable of achieving it. You are helpless and incapable of getting what you want.

WORTHLESSNESS: Belief that you do not deserve the desired goal because of who you are, because of something you did, or because of something you haven't done.

Now, go back to the list from the four categories above and label them where they fall in to these three categories.

Now that you are beginning to generate your limiting belief statements and you have written these limiting belief statements down on the left side of your paper. Now on the right side of the paper, directly across from the appropriate limited belief statement, write the new positive belief statement that answers the question, "What do you want instead of this?" This should be done for all the limiting belief statements once you get the hang of writing what you do want. For example: "I want people to appreciate my gifts, talents, abilities, time, and energy." Or "I want to experience knowing that I am enough, and I am compensated for my value with all the money I need."

Next, once you have your new belief statement written down, ask yourself, "Can it get any better? Can it be more meaningful?" If so, then rewrite it.

To be a compelling statement that you can use to hardwire into your neurology, it must satisfy these five criteria:

Must be in the first person (use the pronoun "I")

Must be in present tense

Must be positively stated

Short (as short as possible but complete)

Meaningful (juicy)

That gets you to your new, juicy belief statement. There are brain balances you can do to synchronize your new belief with a whole brain state. Through entrainment, (meaning to incorporate into), you can sync your new belief system into the neural networks of your body-mind by sitting meditation, active meditation, by a simple Brain Balance Method or the Energy Gateway Visualization. Let's start the process of getting your body (your physiology) trained or in synchronicity with your mind.

Sitting Meditation—This is your typical meditation style where your focus is on your new belief statement. If you have a meditation practice you can just incorporate this into your current meditation method. Also, you could use some of Dr. Joe Dispenza's guided meditations to deepen the repetitiveness of exposure to the new belief statement.

Active Meditation:

This could be a walking meditation and holding the intention of your new belief statement. You could also repeat and hold the intention of your new belief statement while performing Tai Chi energy stabilizing postures or yoga poses.

Therefore, the first aspect of creating change is to change your state. When we say we are feeling sad, we are actually in a "state" of sadness. If you are feeling happy, then we can say you are in a "state" of happiness. If you change your state, you change your physiology. The best way to change your state, thus your physiology (body), is through movement. This is literally your body position. Walking meditation, Tai Chi, and yoga are all ways of movement to create change. Movement in any form will not allow you to stay in the current state of being in which you hold your limited beliefs. An example is if you are depressed, you notice you are slumped, shoulders rounded, dragging your feet when you walk and your head is held down. Then to change your state, stand up straight, hold your head high, pick up your feet, walk with a spring in your step, put a smile on your face, and see if you can stay depressed. It won't be able to happen.

Movement in this simple form has changed your state and your physiology. So, find the state of how you would feel and move if you were truly holding this new belief statement in your body-mind, and how you might think, act, and move if you believed this way. Practice every day, or multiple times per day, synchronizing, acting in this way, rehearsing this way. This process will begin to integrate this new physiology with this new mindset, belief statement.

Brain Balance Method:

The easiest method is to hold the new belief statement while holding ankles crossed, and arms crossed with fingers of the hands interlinked in front of you. This is commonly called a Cook's Hookup.

Through balancing in a whole brain state, we desensitize the original triggers (signals) from our environment or our past that remind us of our habitual state of being. This allows us to move past our limiting belief and we begin to accumulate new triggers (signals) from our environment that allow us to expand into our rewritten beliefs (new state of being) and thus our new behaviors.

We can, in a face-to-face coaching session, check the congruency of a belief between the conscious, super-conscious, and subconscious mind to see if there is an imbalance. We can't do that in this exercise; however, you can let go of the belief causing the imbalance. Then rewrite this belief as best you can and rewire the belief through identifying and clarifying your statements and setting up supportive strategies that will begin to balance the brain in a whole brain state. By doing this, it will allow there to be congruent agreement between the conscious, super-conscious, and subconscious, which allows change to occur and behavior to shift.

Energize the Gateways Visualization:

One last method would be to repeat and hold your new belief statement in your mind and do the Energize the Gateways Visualization that was described earlier. This will allow you to energize all of the systems in your body to this new state of being. You may notice as you are doing it that energy might get sluggish or stuck in a gateway. It would be appropriate at that point to do the 7 Gateway Therapies associated with that gateway until you feel the full natural flow of the gateway as it pertains to this specific new belief statement.

Our strategy is a process of rehearsal that we ultimately do to create new perceptions. Select a new perception, and then determine what belief you would need to support that perception. Then, work backward to what attitude you would need to emotionally embody that new belief. Then progress to what thoughts and feelings you would need to experience to support your new attitude. Then rehearse it many times to hard wire it into the subconscious program.

We are always telling our stories to others as well as to ourselves. These stories are our ongoing dialogue with what is and what we believe is happening around us. Stories are filled with emotion and often drama. Emotion is energy. *It is important to decide where you want to expend your energy. It is equally as critical to decide that you do not want to store imprints that will fester.* Many of us use our energy by telling disempowering stories about life and our role in it.

Your biography is not your destiny; your decisions are your destiny.

We are defined by the stories we tell ourselves. The question then becomes, is your story empowering your life or is it hindering you? Learning to make your stories an authentic expression of who you really are and not letting the stories you tell yourself on the inside be crafted by your inner-saboteur are important in managing your state, strategies, and self-esteem. You are a unique and awesome person. Make your stories, especially the internal ones, inspired and powerful.

Exercise: Smashing the Anger

This particular exercise has been a favorite of mine for a number of years. It is best used for the really hot emotions, such as anger, resentment, frustration, or disgust. It's actually quite an easy and fun process. Here's how it goes.

Go to your local convenience store and buy at least one large bag of ice cubes. Then, take the bag of ice to a place where you feel you can be free to totally express yourself without interruption and can be as loud as you need to be. This could be somewhere in the country where there are large rocks, a place where there is a brick or cement block wall—your own unfinished basement, for instance.

When you find your special place, open the bag of ice cubes. Reach in and grab one or two or a handful of ice cubes. Holding them in your hand, look deeply into the cubes and see whatever it is that is pissing you off ("miffed" from our earlier notes), has pushed your resentment button, or has you disgusted. Then, holding that picture, thought, or image in the ice cubes, throw them as hard as you can at the wall or tree or immovable object that will take the brunt of your emotion. As you do this, let go! Fun, huh!

Now, reach in and get some more ice cubes and see the same image or maybe even one that is more charged than the last and throw those cubes so they shatter. Let go again as you hear the ice cubes smashing. Continue this and let the emotion continue to escape. Let all of your feelings emerge and metaphorically move them out of your body through your arm. As the ice cubes shatter, allow the emotions to shatter as well. As the ice cubes melt, allow the emotions to melt away also.

This is a great process and a powerful one for really "bringing up the stuff." I know in my practice I have had some one baggers as well as some two and three baggers, depending on the level and intensity of emotion that surfaces. Good luck and have fun.

P.S. It is very satisfying to the heart to be able to walk away from this session and let all of the emotion that you have released just melt away on the ground. Get the picture? Good.

Exercise: Emotional Tapping and Integration

Integrative Tapping Method and the Four Master Freedom Points

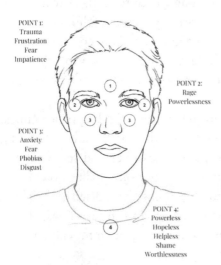

Four Master Freedom Points

POINT 1:
Trauma
Frustration
Fear
Impatience

POINT 2:
Rage
Powerlessness

POINT 3:
Anxiety
Fear
Phobias
Disgust

POINT 4:
Powerless
Hopeless
Helpless
Shame
Worthlessness

Tapping methods have been around for quite some time and are very effective at changing the energy in the body in a time of need. Many times throughout our life, we will be triggered by a memory or a circumstance and those automatic, subconscious programs take over our experience. Once we realize we are in the clutches of this emotional takeover of our otherwise peaceful life, it is often too late to derail that program.

This episode will make our experience less than fun and will limit our possibilities.

With this in mind, it is always good to have a quick and easy method to down grade the emotional storm erupting and return our body, mind, and spirit to a more peaceful and powerful state of being. It is this peaceful and powerful place from which we want to create our experience in life. This state is what allows us to have the response-ability to produce the life we want.

Historically, the acupuncture meridians have been used to alter and normalize energy in the body. The thought is that Chi energy flows continuously through the meridian channels of the body. This flow of energy allows the proper bio-energetic information for maintaining proper regulation of body functions to continue unimpeded. If there is anything that creates stagnation or blockage of this energy flow in the body, then symptoms result.

The original people most responsible for the use of acupoints for psychological problems were Dr. George Goodheart, DC, and Dr. John Diamond, MD. Also, psychologist Roger Callahan was one of the first to develop a psychological treatment based on protocols using 14 specific acupuncture points. Dr. Scott Walker, DC, made popular the connection of the spine, meridians and the body in treatment for psychological events, issues and trauma.

From my study with these and other people who have done work with psychology and meridian-based therapies comes a direct and simple format that can be used by anyone as a tool to turn down or free up the energy around triggered emotions.

This combines information that I have gathered from EFT, TFT, somatoemotional release, NET, neurology and acupuncture. I call it Integrative Tapping, simply because that is what it is. So, let's get to the method.

1. First and foremost is having a specific triggered emotion. Once you have that experience, then you will want to rate the intensity of that emotion on a SUD scale (Subjective Units of Distress Scale) between 1 – 10.

2. Before starting the process, take a moment to remember or create a positive powerful feeling to

replace the empty space left from letting go of the trigger emotion you are currently feeling. Examples may be peace, joy, inspiration, or fulfillment. Take a moment to remember a time when you actually felt this feeling and feel it now for just a moment. Then return your focus to the trigger emotion and continue with the process.

3. Keep your focus on the trigger emotion, trigger issue, and the trigger to incorporate integrative breathing, deep relaxed breaths in and out at equal capacity.

4. The first point to tap in slow repetition is the area between the eyebrows and just above the bridge of the nose, which is just below the area commonly known as the third eye. This point includes the pineal reflex point, the origin of the bladder meridian, and is a reflex center for the prefrontal cortex of the brain. It is a releasing point for trauma, frustration, fear, and impatience. As you begin tapping, allow yourself to focus on the issue or emotion, not the tapping, with relaxed breathing and stating the following:

"It's OKAY for me to let go of this feeling of (insert the emotion or issue) now."

5. Next you will tap on the point at the outside of the eye on the side of the temple. It is a gallbladder point and reflex area for the limbic system, the area of the brain where all emotion is processed. It is a releasing point for rage and powerlessness. Begin tapping with relaxed breathing and state the following:

"I am actually SAFE, letting go of this feeling of (insert the emotion or issue)."

6. Then tapping at the area underneath the eye directly on the cheekbone, which is the point for the beginning of the stomach meridian, this releasing

point focuses on anxiety, fear, phobias, and disgust. At this area, while breathing and tapping, state the following:

"I give myself PERMISSION to totally and completely love and accept myself, even when I feel this feeling of (insert the emotion or issue)."

"I give myself PERMISSION to let go of this feeling of (insert the emotion or issue) now."

7. Now tapping the area where the collarbone and the sternum meet, the notch or V at your neck, this is the point on the meridian system for the kidney (K27). It is the releasing point for powerless, hopeless, helpless, shame, and worthlessness. The K27 point is the association point for all of the meridians and the organs they represent. This tapping allows release from all meridians and organs in the body. At this area breathing and tapping state the following:

"I allow myself the FREEDOM to let go of this feeling of (insert the emotion or issue), and all shock, trauma or conflict, from the present or past, associated with this feeling of (insert the emotion or issue), and I do it now."

8. At this point, you will bring all of your fingertips together in the region over your heart space. All the fingertips together bring brain reflex points and the points of the lung, large intestine, pericardium, and heart meridians together for integration. Now focus your attention on the inspiring or peaceful feeling that you created at the beginning of the process. Taking in at least five deep relaxing breaths and allow yourself to deeply feel the peace, joy, inspiration, or fulfillment you have imagined.

9. End by speaking the descriptive word of the feeling that you are experiencing: Peace. Joy. Fulfillment.

This process is very effective and is remarkable at bringing the SUD scale rating down on an emotion at the time you are experiencing it. Best results are to return later and explore the many aspects of that emotion, situation, or circumstance through the Creative Imaging Method or other methods available. However, it is effective in quickly returning you to a path of conscious choice and emotional balance that is empowering. And you can accomplish it just about anywhere—in your car, at work, in your office or bathroom, or while on a walk to expend energy and find calm.

Short Tapas Acupressure Technique (STAT)

Tapas Acupressure Technique, TAT, was developed by Elizabeth Tapas Fleming, an acupuncturist. This method being shared here is not TAT, nor is it meant to imply that it is in anyway connected to the Tapas Technique. To benefit fully from TAT, you need to either be trained as a TAT professional or work with someone who is. If you go to her website, tatlife.com, the certified TAT professionals and trainers listed on her website are happy to help you.

For purposes of this book in clearing emotions, we will use a short version similar to some of the aspects of TAT; however, the holding points have changed for STAT and we will do a bit of a different program as far as the steps involved in the emotional stabilization that we are seeking as a self-help tool.

With one hand, lightly touch the tip of the thumb and the tip of the little finger to an area on each side of the bridge of the nose and just where the inner corner of the eye meets the bridge of the nose. Place the tip of the middle finger at the point midway between the inner aspects of the eyebrows. Place the ring and index fingers on the forehead just above the mid portion of the eyebrow, respectively, in the area known as the Bennett Points. All five fingers of the holding or pose hand should now be gently touching the face, with the three fingers in line on the forehead.

Now, place your other hand on the back of your head, in the area of the occipital bone of the cranium, just above where the top of the neck and the bottom aspect of the head meet at that slight upside-down U indentation. This is the occipital area and is also the visual representation area of the brain. The palm of the hand cradles the base of your skull. Both hands should be resting gently, and no significant pressure is necessary.

You can rest your arms at any time during a step or between steps. Eyes can be open or closed, and either hand can be in front or back, whichever is more comfortable, or you can switch hands during the process if needed.

Rarely will the feeling you are working at decreasing get stronger during the process; if, however, the feeling does get stronger, continue with the STAT pose and focus your attention on the intention set out in the step that you are doing at the time. Don't put your attention on getting more and more into those feelings that are increasing. Your feelings usually become more peaceful within a few minutes.

Note: For children or a person who can't do this pose for themselves, you can cover the points with your own hands, front and back. I recommend doing this pose on everything, from emotional difficulties, pain, discomfort, traumatic memories, as well as allergies.

At the beginning of a session, it is helpful to hold an intention that the healing you are about to do will benefit all parts of you, everyone involved, and all points of view you have ever held. With each step, hold the STAT pose and put your attention on the thought expressed in that step, for about a minute or until you're done. Indicators that you're done can include a sigh, an energy release, a yawn, or simply a feeling of being done. Some people don't notice any change and simply sit with each step for about a minute. Children may only need a few seconds for each step.

Stat Finger and Hand Placement Diagram

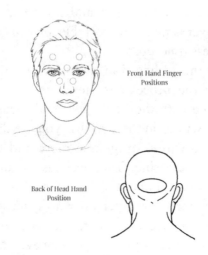

Front Hand Finger
Positions

Back of Head Hand
Position

Step One: The Problem

It is important to know that when you're working with STAT on an incident from the past, it is not necessary nor is it recommended to relive or re-experience past events in order for them to be healed. In fact, you don't even have to specifically describe the event. You can simply refer to the event as "this", for instance you would state, "<u>This</u> happened." However, if it helps you to be more detailed, you may want to say, " _____ happened." Just filling in the blank with your description, such as <u>"the accident happened"</u> or <u>"the time that I got angry and yelled at my child happened"</u>.

Step Two: The Opposite of the Problem

Step 2 is a companion to step 1 and is infinitely variable. Keep in mind that you put your attention on the opposite of the problem; you are not being asked to believe the statement, just simply be with it or the possibility.

Use the following statement, "_____ happened, it's over, and I'm okay. I can relax now."

This is using the concept of "I'm okay" in a universal sense, where the eternal part of you is unaffected by the events of this life and forever okay. For an ongoing circumstance or situation, you can say: "_____ (this) is happening and I'm okay."

Step Three: The Issues in the Tissues

Emotions, stressful biochemistry, and less than positive thoughts can and do get stored in the tissues of the body. They can be neurologically tied or anchored to the environment where the event happened, a specific house, city, or season, even a specific group, or race of people. Each person stores these memories differently. You don't need to be aware of all of the places where the event or problem is linked. You just need to be open to the intention of any anchor or neurological linkage being completely healed.

To do this step you put your attention on this statement, "All the places in my mind, body, and life where this has been stored are healing now."

Step Four: Shame Resilience

In her book, *Daring Greatly*, Brené Brown speaks to the concept of shame resilience. What is meant by shame resilience is the ability to practice authenticity when we experience shame, to move through the experience without sacrificing our values, and to come out on the other side of the shame experience with more courage, compassion, and connection than we had going into it. Shame resilience is about moving from shame to empathy, which is the real antidote to shame. If we can share our story with someone who responds with empathy and understanding, shame can't survive.

People often want to believe that shame is reserved for people who have survived an unspeakable trauma, but this is not true. There are three things you need to know about shame.

1. We all have it; shame is universal and one of the most primitive human emotions that we experience.

2. We're all afraid to talk about shame.

3. The less we talk about shame, the more control it has over our lives.

Shame is the fear of disconnection. We are psychologically, emotionally, cognitively, and spiritually hardwired for connection, love, and belonging. Connection, love, and belonging are why we are here, and it is what gives purpose and meaning to our lives. Shame is the fear of disconnection—it is the fear that something we've done or failed to do, an ideal that we've not lived up to, or a goal that we've not accomplished makes us unworthy of connection. I'm not worthy or good enough for love, belonging, or connection. I'm unlovable. I don't belong. This is what is said to recognize, be aware, reach out through self-compassion and speak to shame.

"I reach out to connect."
"I am worthy."
"I'm lovable."
"I belong."
"I am enough."

Step Five: Integration

This step is for completely integrating the healing from this session into your bioenergy field. "This healing is completely integrated now, with my grateful thanks." That's it.

It is amazingly simple, yet elegantly effective. The first few times you do this process, you may want to rate the intensity of the problem before the session, using the SUD scale of 0 – 10, with 0 indicating "no stress" and 10 indicating "the worst possible." Then rate how you feel when you focus on the event, trauma or emotion at the end of the session. Compare your before and after ratings.

Of course, the real test for the effectiveness of STAT in your life will be the changes you see. Sometimes you may feel immediate big shifts. Other times the changes might be much more subtle. Most importantly, all of these changes contribute to living a happier life.

Meditations

The mind interrupts the process of manifesting things by sound, which is used in some meditations. It is the resonating energy we produce to achieve disruption of the disruption. One of the most beneficial things we can create for our body, mind, and spirit is peacefulness. I have found that starting the day with meditation and an intention for good to happen will set a positive tone for my daily experiences. Granted, many things throughout the day will compete for space in your mind and awareness. Most of these are distractions that will, bit by bit, peck away at your peace and leave you devoid of focus and bliss by the end of the day. Part of the concept of unpacking your backpack at the end of the day is to let go of all those energies you have picked up throughout your day's journey. Two very powerful and impactful meditations I recommend are the Morning Manifestation and the Evening Release.

Morning Manifestation Meditation

The sound used in the Morning Manifestation Meditation is *Ahh*, which is a primal sound that is part of all creation. It is the energy of creation itself. It is the ancient sound and vibration of manifestation. Ahh is associated with joy. It's the sound used to create getting a clear and focused image of what you want to create or manifest for the day. When we say, Ahh, it invokes joy, which invokes creation and the manifestation of your desired intention. *Ahh. Ahhh. Ahhhhh.*

Ahh is the link between the Foundation Gateway, root chakra, the area of the body or energy matrix associated with creation, and the Vision Gateway, third eye, the area of visioning for our mind and spirit. All the distracting thoughts of the mind will pull energy away from your creation process. The morning meditation will let the mind melt away and allow your idea, thought, or intention to flow into the material world or lovingly toward another person.

Begin this meditation by finding a comfortable place to sit, preferably where you can make noise, feel uninhibited, and be uninterrupted for approximately 20 minutes. As you focus your mind on what you want to create or send out into the world, close your eyes and settle your breathing. As you inhale, focus your mind on your intention, your manifestation. As you let your air out, relax your throat and let the word 'Ahh' carry this intention from you out to the Universe. Do this, unafraid of being heard.

Think about the things you would like to create in the world from the place of this positive manifestation. Maybe you would like to create a divine relationship. Perhaps you want to establish a new empowering belief or perception in your life. Maybe you are ready to create a new aspect of your personality, a new habit, or a new behavior. Perhaps you would like to create a change around your job, your relationship, or your creativity. Perhaps you would like to be lighter, let go of some weight. If you would like to open to this energy of healing then, do it now.

Maybe you have had a sense of scarcity in your life and you would like to create more abundance or security around you. Perhaps you would like to let go of stress, high blood pressure, or anxiety in your life to create more peace, balance, and a feeling of oneness with nature.

Whatever it is that you would like to manifest, I urge you to suspend all doubt and be willing every morning to begin your day with the practice of the Ahh Morning Manifestation Meditation. During the meditation, allow yourself to imagine and feel the flow of energy in your body between the Foundation Gateway, root chakra (your lower abdomen or pelvis) and the Vision Gateway, third eye center (between your eyes at the forehead). After a consistent practice of this meditation, you may begin to notice your intention in meditation will begin to reveal the manifestation of that intention in your life.

I suggest in this meditation that from midway to the end of the meditation you insert your own or the following affirmations. You may want to start and finish with one of these affirmations, or you may want to put more than two affirmations in a meditation session. For example:

At the beginning of the meditation, say in an affirmative, confident, and focused tone, *I am love, light and happiness.*

Then inhale, saying '*Ahh*' as you breathe out, mentally sending out into the world the energy of the affirmation or intention.

Then with your focus on the intention of your particular meditation that day, holding that feeling and thought, you can breathe in, with the focus on the feeling and thought of your intention, saying *'Ahh'* as you breathe out. Repeat this process for 10 breaths and repeat more cycles of 10 breaths for as long as you want to stay in meditation. This allows you to make your meditation time as short or as long you choose.

When you get to the end of your meditation, you want to close with the next phrase saying, in an affirmative, confident and focused tone, *I know in each moment I am free to choose.*

Inhaling, say, *'Ahh'*, as you are exhaling, mentally sending out into the world the energy of this affirmation or intention.

Repeat this process over the next few weeks with each of the following affirmations, intentions or make up your own. Go for it! Here are some examples:

I realize I'm always free to let go and observe my life.

I know that my infinite self is always ready to rise beyond the world I experience with my senses.

My past is nothing more than the trail that I've left behind.

My past has no more meaning than the meaning I choose to give it.

My present and future are determined by the energy that I generate in each of my present moments.

I rid myself of my doubt by remembering there is a powerful perspective I can create for everything that happens in my life.

The more I listen, the more profound the silence becomes.

I am totally responsible for my perspective in response to all that happens in my life.

I know that the very essence of my being is love.

I know that I live in an ocean of love that surrounds me constantly.

I let go of my judgments because they prevent me from seeing the good that lies beyond appearances.

I know I can connect my mind with the infinite ocean of love and be guaranteed peace at any moment.

I know that I am whole. I need not chase after anything in order to be complete.

I will be in this day with the highest intention for the highest good of all.

I will radiate integrity, truth, love, peace, and joy from my Infinite Self for the collective good of all.

This is a morning meditation. Each of these affirmations is a powerful indication of what you will be able to manifest in your own material world. You are taking the sound of creation and whispering your intention throughout the entire Universe. It is the sound of the creative energy of the Universe or your Source that has been handed down, in all languages, since the beginning of time.

You are essentially creating a sound wave to carry your intention, your positive manifestation, through the expanse of time. As it moves through the air, it will attract, collect, and transform energies that will begin the process of bringing your intention into a material manifestation in your life.

Make it meaningful, make it juicy, and let go without getting attached to the outcome. Notice when and how it shows up for you. Then celebrate!!

Evening Release Meditation

The *Ahh* meditation (Morning Manifestation Meditation) focuses on the manifestation of your desires through the sound of '*Ahh*'. The Evening Release Meditation allows you to let go of your desires and to experience joy and gratitude for being who you are and what you are. It allows you to let go of all that you have accumulated in the way of fear, doubt and burden from the day.

The sound *Ahh* is the first sound of creation. The sound '*Ohm*' is the sound of peace, harmony, joy, and happiness in your life. It is the sound of serenity. It's the sound that you want to go to sleep with every night. In this meditation, as in the Ahh meditation, we are using sound vibration and resonance to bring you to the serene inner bliss that is your Infinite Self, that place inside yourself where you let go of what you want to manifest and instead put all your energy into being grateful, taking on a spirit of gratitude.

The goal of life is to love and to find love within yourself, to unconditionally love yourself and to be grateful for the infinite, divine and loving soul that you are.

Get into a comfortable position, where you can make some sound aloud and feel uninhibited. Now, breathe in and say the sound '*Ohm*' as you breathe out.

Feel the serenity. Inhale, and say the sound of '*Ohm*' as you exhale.

Be thankful for all that you are. Breathe in and say '*Ohm*' as you breathe out.

Be thankful for all that you have. Inhale, and say '*Ohm*' as you exhale.

Unconditionally love your Infinite and Sacred Self. Breathe in, and say '*Ohm*' as you breathe out.

Love and accept yourself just as you are. Inhale, and say '*Ohm*' as you exhale.

Breathe in and repeat '*Ohm*' as you breathe out.

Then with your attention on gratitude, hold that feeling and thought, breathe in holding the feeling of gratitude, say 'Ohm' and breathe out. Repeat this process for 10 breaths and repeat more cycles of 10 breaths as many times as you like, depending on how long you want to continue the meditation. It is good to begin the meditation with an affirmation and end the meditation with an affirmation. You can choose one offered here or make up your own. You can change the affirmations and see how they feel to you and then use the ones that feel appropriate for you at the time.

Repeat this process with each of the following affirmations, intentions or make up your own. Go for it! Here are some examples:

I am unique in the Universe.

I am peace, love and acceptance.

I am powerful in my stillness.

I claim my power to make change in my life.

I release all chaos and constricted energy from my life.

I release all blocks to the perfect flow in my life.

I rest in my acceptance of myself, my wholeness, and my faith in the divine rightness of all life.

Know that when you go to sleep you will rest peacefully and be blanketed in love, surrounded by the infinite ocean of love that permeates all around you, only to rise again to the Ahh meditation, and another day of positive manifesting.

Epilogue

What we learned throughout this book is that the Health Code reveals a form of "Bio-Symbolism" or "Bio-Cognition" that can help us to realize what traumas hold us from fully being ourselves. Once we are aware of the location of blocks, tension, or discomfort in our bodies, we can bring awareness to what Health Code we might want to create for the best resolution of this limitation, then free ourselves to embrace the alignment of our body-mind for optimal wellness.

As you learned new concepts through this book, you may have experienced different feelings, possibly body tension or uneasiness. If so, what you are experiencing is a normal response to being reminded of things that may be imbalanced energy patterns from the past. It is actually not uncommon to have a couple of possible reactions. You may have noticed immediate responses like tightness in your chest, unexplained pain in a body region, or clearing of your throat. On the other hand, you may not have noticed anything while reading, but once finished, felt a slight twinge in your gut, a memory surface of an old auto accident, a reminder of a breakup with a loved one, or another traumatic time from your past. It is important to understand that almost any response you might have is an activation of the energy pattern you experienced during an original overwhelming event somewhere in your life. It is that place where you let some event in your energy flow get blocked and stored, and that past disharmony is now triggered in your human energy field. The reason it is important to pay attention to these feelings is first for your own healing. It is also important to be aware of how it feels when these feelings arise so you can carry that experience into your healing work with others. It will give you a level of understanding and compassion for their process that will enhance their healing experience.

It is exciting and curious to understand that any symptoms that you have had or are currently experiencing appear so that you may explore the emotional imbalance associated with the overwhelm or trauma. The symptoms or bio-symbols can and will disappear when the trauma is healed. In order to heal the trauma, we need to learn to trust the messages, and the insights our body is giving us. You can then teach your patients to begin the process of trusting the messages that come for them. These biosymbols are appearing at an appropriate time to reframe your view of these activated symptoms. You and your clients can begin to be grateful that your bodies are sending messages letting you know that healing needs to happen.

When there is unresolved trauma there is a compulsion to repeat the actions that caused the problem in the first place. Some people consider this a type of karma. Triggering of these traumas may be played out in intimate relationships, work situations, repetitive accidents, injuries, mishaps, or in other seemingly random events. They may also appear in the form of chronic bodily symptoms or in repetitive dreams. This is our body-mind trying to work out a resolution. Most of us are totally unaware of this connection. It is all played out subconsciously, just beneath our awareness.

The good news is that we (or our clients) don't have to completely relive the experience of an event to heal from it. Visiting one's charged energy around a trauma is different than reliving it. Because trauma happens primarily on an energetic level, the memories we have of overwhelming events are stored as disharmonies in our bodies. When we access or help our clients access these memories through exploring the Health Code, we can begin to feel them and begin to discharge the instinctive survival energy of the original event. Shake it off. Utilizing our ability to feel and become body aware is a way of paying attention to our internal wake-up calls. If we learn to listen to these calls, learn how to increase the awareness of our bodies through some of the methods in this book, then we have the power to use these messages and can begin to heal our traumas as well as our lives. Body awareness is something we want to cultivate and make an integral part of our lives because when we are disconnected from our bodies, we can't be fully present. Living in a body-aware way gives all of us a sense of aliveness and purpose in all areas of our lives. It gives us access to our Health Code for wellness in body, mind and life.

If you or your patients notice that you are avoiding certain feelings, people, situations and places in your life, then you are living in a disconnected manner. This disconnection is limiting our choices in life and you can find a way to heal your life, and your patients' lives, with the exercises in this book. It is important to understand that living in disconnection may be limiting the experiences in life that ultimately would highlight our excellence or our genius. The world cannot afford this loss of connection to ourselves, to our bodies, to our families, to others and to the possibilities around us.

This is where I would encourage you to take time every day or at least every week to align your body and mind to your Health Code. I would encourage you to ask your clients and patients to do the same. Follow this process. Take time to align your energy with the Health Code by following these steps:

- **Body awareness:** this is the process of breathing and becoming aware of where in the body you are holding tension, discomfort or any unusual sensation. Allow yourself to inhale into it, allow the feeling, embrace the feeling and then exhale and release the tension.

- **Stay open and curious:** as you focus and stay aware of the area of tension in your body allow yourself to stay open and curious about what feelings, emotions or thoughts are being revealed within this state of tension. What could possibly be going on mentally and emotionally in your life right now to generate this tension in your body?

- **Heal the gateway:** once you know where the tension is, go to your body charts and find the gateway associated with this area of the body or the organ. See if you can find the most appropriate emotion associated with this area or gateway. Assist the release from the gateway with an appropriate essential oil on the gateway point or experience the yoga pose, place a stone on the gateway point or tap on the gateway point.

- **Releasing the emotion:** As you release the tension with your breath, you release your attachment to the emotions you are experiencing. You are letting go of the charge, or the disruptive energy of the emotions. In addition, say the mantra for the gateway and breathe and release more of the tension or emotion.

- **Create a plan:** create a plan to change your perspective, belief or attitude about the situation that is triggering your tension and emotional disharmony. Plan to change your actions so that you can let go of the cycle of rumination with this issue or trauma within yourself that keeps this tension chronically in your body.

- **Journal or talk:** after you have cleared the issue, and your energy feels more balanced, write in a journal about your breakthroughs, or talk to someone you love and trust about the discoveries you make along the way with each experience.

- **Tap it out:** allow yourself in the interim of the change that takes place over the next days, weeks, months to be kind and compassionate to yourself. When the old patterns try to return, or an inkling of it returns, tap out the residual emotions through one of the exercises in this book or another tapping method of your choice.

The whole point of this book is to hopefully open your awareness, recognition, and intuition to the fact that you possess the answers to all of your challenges. It is imperative that you be a teacher in your healing practice and let your clients know that they possess the answers to all of their challenges as well. Let them know that the answers are inside of you, not outside of you. It does require your commitment to explore and trust your inner guidance in conjunction with inner knowing. It requires that you believe in yourself and that you elevate your self-esteem. This is your life. Don't sell yourself short. Take the insights your body is offering and trust the part of you that knows there is truth and love in the knowledge, hunch, or coincidence of thoughts and experience. Use this information to give yourself permission to be honest with yourself, to love yourself enough to find the courage to realize your birthright.

I hope that you begin to hear the whispering of your inner knowing of your body and the bodies of your patients. The Health Code gives all of you guidance where the healing can start today. Through the healing experiences of your life, you will be reminded that you are connected to all other forms of life on the planet. Respect our planet and all living forms. I believe that you can begin to enjoy the magnificence of following your inner guidance and intuition. I know that you will begin to see and feel the connectedness of all things. Share your gifts, talents, and abilities with the world. This is why you are here. It is your only assignment; it is your soul purpose.

Thank you for stepping courageously into healing your body and your life. Thank you for expressing the magnificence of who you are! Make your life your message. Live life in harmony with yourself, others, and nature.

References

(In Alphabetical Order)

Brown, Brené. *Daring Greatly, How the Courage to Be Vulnerable Transforms the Way We Live, Love, Parent, and Lead*, Penguin Random House, 2012.

Childre, Doc Lee. Founder, HeartMath Institute. (https://www.heartmath.com)

Chopra, Deepak. *Perfect Health: The Complete Mind/Body Guide*. Three Rivers Press. 1991.

Diamond, John. *Life Energy: Using the Meridians to Unlock Your Emotions*. Paragon House Publishers. 1998.

Flemming, Elizabeth Tapas, Tapas Acupressure Technique. (https://tatlife.com)

Gerber, Richard, MD, *Vibrational Medicine, The #1 Handbook of Subtle-Energy Therapies*, Third Edition, Bear Company, 2001.

Goodheart, George. *Applied Kinesiology*. Touch for Health. 2013.

Hendricks, Gay and Kathleen, The Hendricks Institute. (https://hendricks.com)

Laporte, Danielle. *The Desire Map: A Guide to Creating Goals with Soul*. Sounds True. 2012.

Levine, Peter A. *In an Unspoken Voice: How the Body Releases Trauma and Restores Goodness*. Penguin Random House Publishers. 2010.

Lipton, Bruce H. *The Biology of Belief: Unleashing the Power of Consciousness, Matter and Miracles*. 2016.

McMakin, Carolyn and Oschman, PhD *The Resonance Effect, How Frequency Specific Microcurrent is Changing Medicine,* North Atlantic Books, April 25, 2017.

Parker, Karen Curry. *Understanding Human Design: the New Science of Astrology: Discover Who You Really Are.* Hierophant Publishing. 2013.

Sarno, John. *The Divided Mind: The Epidemic of Mind Body Disorders.* HarperCollins Publishers. 2006.

Williams, Robert. Psych-K, 2015. (https://psych-k.com)

Acknowledgments

With the discovery, treatment, and recovery from cancer, I finished this book. That was one of the hardest and yet most rewarding processes I have ever voluntarily taken on in my life. The amount of focus, effort and time to write and research this book was at times overwhelming yet rewarding to put these concepts together. It required me to draw from my past years of experience in a busy practice, from workshops, teachers, mentors and the evolution of science validating the work of healers and innovators in health and wellness.

I learned through this process many things about myself, which is always a good thing, even if difficult to face, but also learned about how much it takes to put a project like this together. Writing a book is a thing many of us talk about and have the intention to do. Intention, like most intention, is a fickle beast that plays with our minds on a regular basis. But that aside, what a wonderful exercise and a privilege to have had the opportunity to experience. This could never have been realized without a village of people to support, encourage and well . . . put up with me during this process. My family being the first in line for praise. I am grateful beyond measure for their resilience to allow me to be sometimes absent physically while tapping away on my computer keyboard, but mostly me being sometimes mentally absent, while words, phrases, structures, concepts would arise unexpectedly and in random sequences throughout my days and nights.

A special expression of gratitude goes to my dear friend Michelle, who kept persistently encouraging me to continue to write and finally to take me by the hand and actually get the book published. I am grateful to GracePoint Matrix for publishing this book, Michelle Vandepas and Karen Curry Parker, who were more than gracious and generous to do so. I am honored and encouraged to acknowledge the expertise of my professional editors Heather Hilliard and Shauna Hardy who without them this book would not have happened. They made me a better writer throughout their coaching. Also, acknowledgment goes to Gracie at GracePoint Publishing for being my books project manager and getting through the final stages of putting this out in the world. My ability to even think and somewhat act like a writer must be credited to my first creative writing instructor Jane Hilberry, who actually got me started on this idea of writing about my healing experiences many moons ago. It was her early guidance and encouragement I have always reflected back on through this process.

There is a deep gratefulness for the encouragement of many of my coaching clients and clinic patients who over the years have encouraged me to write about the healing experiences we have all been able to experience. There are feelings of love and acknowledgment for all of the students that I have had an opportunity to share many of these methods with. Grateful that many of these same people prompted me to put this material into a book. Fortunate and grateful for all of my colleagues who ask me questions, ask for advice in practice and in their own healing, so as to help as many people as possible with tapping into their own healer within.

I want to recognize all of the pioneers and innovators that I have had the blessing of being taught, mentored and just generally hanging out with for the last 40 years of my life. They are from many different walks of life and many different aspects of healing, from my own profession, Dr. Joe Dispenza, Dr. John DeMartini, Dr. Scott Walker, Dr. Alan Beardall, Dr. George Goodheart, Dr. John Brimhall, Dr. Ted Morter, Dr. Louisa Williams, as well as many of my professors that enlightened my thinking in ways it is too difficult to articulate.

It is imperative to acknowledge and recognize those outside of my profession for their tireless work to help humanity and to educate the world about healing in a non-mainstream manner. Their innovative ideas and methods have become the actual fabric of my being over the years. These incredible pioneers have made an impact on the world that will live on forever: Dr. Bruce Lipton, Gay and Kathleen Hendricks, Dr. Richard Gerber, MD, James

Oschmann. PhD, Dr. Thomas Meyers, Dr. Peter Levine, Leon and Mary Overbay, and Tony Robbins. I am grateful for what I've learned from them about managing my own life and am grateful they have given me a more empowering way to look at the world around me and to live fully in the world.

At the top of my eternally grateful list is my family of origin and for the environment they created for me growing up so that I could find myself. My mother and father, Margie and Charlie Daugherty, for their presence in my life, and their examples, values and positive influence. To my friends, coaches, and brothers Chuck, Terry, and David Daugherty, who always encouraged me. My brother Chuck provided expansive experiences for me in my life that allowed me to grow and have a bigger perspective on possibilities. My brother, Terry, was an inspiration from which I learned to balance between drive, ambition and compassion for others. My brother, David, especially throughout his life, was my confidant in life to keep me on track, push me when I needed it and to be the voice of understanding in my life when I was confused and off track. Unfortunately, this year, 2020 was a tough year for so many, but especially my own family. My Father passed this year just shy of his birthday at the age of 101. Both my brother, David, and my brother Chuck passed this year as well. All within a few days to a few months of each other. My beloved Mother passed in 2010 and all of us boys banded together to carry on her loving spirit. I would have loved to have shared the completion of this book with them. I wish they could have been alive to see the fruits of this project. I know they are present in and around me now. It is such an honor to have all of my brother's families still a strong presence in my life on a daily basis. Thank you for your love and guidance.

Always, I am more than grateful for the support, love, understanding and thought-provoking family that surrounds me all of the time. They are so crucial to my own personal growth on a daily basis and always help me see myself better. I could not have accomplished this without their generous support, love and encouragement. My incredible beloved, Susan Daugherty, who is my champion, guidepost, and eternal love. To my children Micah Sutton, my son Matthew Daugherty, my daughter-in-law

Leah Daugherty, my son Ryan Daugherty, daughter in law Angie Daugherty, and all six of my grandchildren Sylvia, Miles, Wynn, Sophie, Farrah, and Lucy. I hope someday to have left a positive legacy for this tribe of amazing people.

About the Author

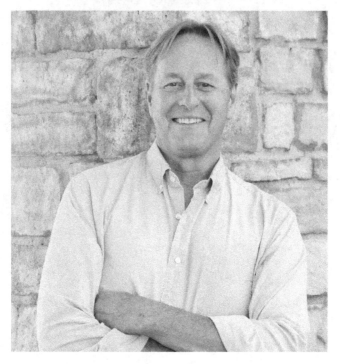

Dr. John Daugherty is a practicing chiropractor, but his patients prefer to call him a healer. He is a student of many methodologies including Bio-Energy medicine, Functional and Integrative medicine, and human behavior training to include the Hendricks Institute and Neuro-Emotional and Somato-Emotional Therapies.

With his many years of study and practice and his constant quest to learn more about universal laws and principles and how they affect overall health, Dr. Daugherty developed The Health Code, a guide to assist everyone in reaching their authentic self while gaining peak wellness in both body and mind.

**Find out more and download more resources at
TheHealthCodeBook.com**

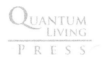

Discover more great books at GracePointPublishing.com

CPSIA information can be obtained
at www.ICGtesting.com
Printed in the USA
JSHW041929060721
16617JS00003B/15